Cancer

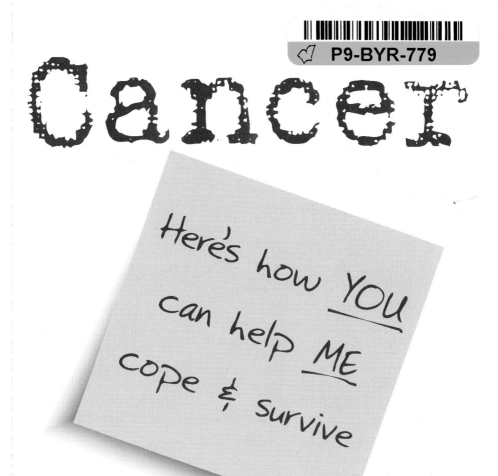

Here's how <u>YOU</u> can help <u>ME</u> cope & survive

A practical handbook on
strengthening the bond
between cancer patients,
family and friends

By Joy Erlichman Miller, Ph.D & Monica Vest Wheeler
with Diane Cullinan Oberhelman

Cancer: Here's how YOU can help ME cope & survive

ISBN 0-9759875-1-8

2

Cover design by Gina Edwards

Net proceeds of this book will be donated to the Cancer Center for Healthy Living in Peoria, Illinois; Kids Konnected and other cancer-related programs.

BF Press
P.O. Box 3065
Peoria, IL 61612-3065

Contact us online and order additional books at:
www.cancerhelpbook.com

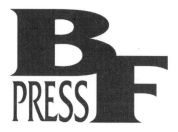

What's inside

3

4

The many reasons why we needed this book

Preface by Diane Cullinan Oberhelman

Diagnosed with an aggressive form of breast cancer in July 1995, I was only 36 years old. With no family history of cancer, this was quite a shock.

Amidst the whirlwind of doctors, surgery, chemotherapy, stem cell transplant, radiation and family, I found one of the most distressing parts of the whole experience was how people had difficulty communicating with me. They avoided me, afraid to say the "wrong" thing. Others kept my family and me in their thoughts and prayers, but they could not bring themselves to do anything in person because of the fear of rejection. I also searched for the right things to do and say to make all around me comfortable and at ease. I noticed friends and acquaintances walk to the other side of the street when they would see me coming, out of fear of saying or doing the wrong thing.

What could I do to make *them* feel better? I thought I needed outside guidance and help. Certainly there must be a book or a communication guide that I could purchase that would have the answers. I searched bookstores and on the internet, but I couldn't find what I wanted and needed in the fall of 1995.

Embarrassed, I asked the bookstore clerk to help me find such a book in the cancer or communication sections. My search came up empty. The salesperson and I were both surprised that there was no such book.

> "I noticed friends and acquaintances walk to the other side of the street when they would see me coming out of fear of saying or doing the wrong thing."

I told myself, when I make it through all of this, I am going to write a book to assist cancer patients, their loved ones, friends, co-workers, children and spouses. The book would center on what cancer patients need related to help, support, effective communication and means of coping with the diagnosis.

Needless to say, recovery from my extensive treatment was much more than I could ever imagine. I was in survival mode for many months after the mastectomy, chemotherapy, transplant and radiation. It took all my energy and focus to get through the day, much less think about a book.

In 1997, I gained the strength to look back at my notes from this traumatic experience and started to work on the book. I recognized I needed the assistance of professionals and turned to Dr. Joy Erlichman Miller, who is a renowned author and dear friend. She has written many books and has such a wonderful way with words. She thought the idea was great, and we started on the journey. However, we were both immediately sidetracked due to my challenges at work and Joy's full agenda at her very successful psychotherapy business.

I spoke to many survivors and caregivers, and all concurred enthusiastically that this book was desperately needed. Deter-mined to start the book again, a few years later at one of the support group meetings that my children — Kathleen, Maureen, Alison and Allen — had founded along with Judy Oakford, I ran into Robin and Lenny Unes and their beautiful children. Sadly, they were attending the meetings again because of Robin's recurrence of breast cancer. My heart sank as she told me about her cancer returning with a vengeance.

It was the right moment to tell her about my idea about "the book" and the vision to donate the proceeds to cancer-related causes. Robin was astounded as she was doing the same thing but had felt too weak recently to work on it. We both broke down in tears with amazement that we could possibly be working on what we hoped would be a significant contribution to cancer patients, their families, friends, and anyone who knew a cancer patient and wanted to assist them in any way. Robin and I hugged and agreed that when she felt better, which I was so confident she would, we could collaborate and publish the book to help cancer patients and survivors all over the world.

When my husband, Doug, and I were out of town in May 2003, we came back to learn Robin had died. No! I thought the person

6

who told me must be mistaken, ill-informed and downright wrong! This could not be true! Only after seeing her obituary did I believe it. Such a tragedy.

Later, the book idea came to light again as Joy Erlichman Miller, Lenny Unes and I connected. Coincidentally, Joy had taught Lenny in school years earlier. Robin had left behind a stack of handwritten notes, and Lenny shared those with us. At that time, Joy thought that to make this book reach its full potential, we needed to involve yet another incredible author of fabulous books, Monica Vest Wheeler. I wholeheartedly agreed.

The combination of Joy and Monica is truly a sight to see. They are the most talented writers I have ever witnessed and are dedicated beyond belief. They are so prolific with their words and descriptions. If it were not for their leadership with this book, it would not be here today. They are incredible!

Needless to say, Lenny Unes wanted Robin's words and message to live on through this book. My small part in this journey was more from my personal experience as a survivor and the desire to see this book written, and to see this information shared with those who need it. Joy and Monica have captured the essence of Robin's thoughts and desires, and have created a platform in which cancer patients can learn how to interface with people closest to them and vice versa. They are to be commended. They worked tirelessly and pulled many all-nighters to see this to fruition. They also were committed to seeing that proceeds go to cancer-related causes such as the Cancer Center for Health Living in Peoria and the support group for children, Kids Konnected. These are two incredible ladies.

The three of us would like to dedicate this book to Robin Unes as her contributions in this endeavor will touch so many lives in a very positive way. We feel she has inspired us to finish this important piece of work for you to experience.

"We feel Robin has inspired us to finish this important piece of work for you to experience."

Just one of many

8

Robin Cameron Unes was just one of many individuals who fiercely battled cancer during their lifetime. Most of us have met a Robin somewhere along the way, human beings who persevered and inspired others with their resiliency and plain old courage.

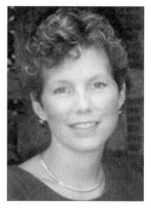

Yes, Robin is but one of the many reasons this book has been compiled. She lost her fight of several years against breast cancer at the age of 38 on May 2, 2003. Until then, Robin had scribbled her thoughts about the unique needs of cancer patients based on her own experiences and those of friends. She brainstormed with fellow soldiers in this campaign against this notorious enemy called cancer. She wanted to do something with this acquired knowledge and insight, something to assist other patients and their loved ones with the struggle, something that would lighten their load.

Unfortunately, Robin did not live long enough to turn that dream into a reality. In 2004, her gracious husband, Leonard Unes II, affectionately called Lenny, wanted Robin's work to continue and came to us asking for our assistance to complete her mission.

We had been influenced by experiences of our own. Diane had battled breast cancer herself, and Joy and Monica had watched loved ones around them confront cancer. With much commitment, enthusiasm and admiration, we decided to give this seedling of an idea a place to grow in our fertile imaginations. The ideas mushroomed, and thus was born this volume, far beyond our original expectations in size and scope.

We are abiding by Lenny's request that this not be a book about *his* Robin, because there are so many other people suffering the pain cancer inflicts. However, you will find some of the thoughts Robin and her friends jotted down throughout this book on pages under the *"Just one of many"* heading. We also felt you should see Robin's smile and read her words on the facing page, a poem that has left an indelible impression upon us. You'll understand immediately why this book was born … because the need, unfortunately, is so great.

Today I Am A Survivor

by Robin Unes

October 1, 1964–May 2, 2003

Yesterday I learned I had cancer,
But today I became a survivor.

Yesterday I was full of worry and stress,
But today I found faith that things will work out.

Yesterday I was angry and mad at the world,
But today I laughed and found humor where I could.

Yesterday I blamed others for the problems that I see,
But today I took charge and helped someone in need.

Yesterday my future seemed so uncertain and sad,
But today I give thanks for each and every day.

Yesterday I was lonely, pushing away family and
    friends,
But today I told them I love them now, tomorrow
    and always.

Yesterday I just had cancer,
But today I became a survivor!

(Inspired by the life and love of Barbara Walvoord)

The secret behind this special book

We want you to use and abuse this book. That's why the pages are perforated and there are spaces to write your thoughts, needs and emotions. This is an *interactive* guidebook that attempts to cure one of the nastiest by-products of cancer: ***The lack of communication between cancer patients/survivors and their family and friends.*** We're focusing on the equally important and vital emotional connection, which reinforces affiliation, love, friendship and human resiliency. Open this book to any page, and you will find some words of encouragement or the right questions to help you address your own concerns, whether you're a patient/survivor, family member or friend. There literally is something for everyone.

The very word *cancer* can shake the most stoic of individuals. *Cancer* or the big *"C"* is a six-letter word or single letter that evokes fear. Our research and respective life experiences have shown us that many cancer patients/survivors have difficulty in asking for assistance, and that many loved ones and friends don't know what to say or do when faced with this horrible news. The American Cancer Society estimates there will be more than 1.3 million new cases diagnosed in 2005, and more than half a million deaths from the disease. And that's not counting the millions of others who still battle cancer, who are in remission, and all who vow to survive every day.

Perhaps the greatest lesson is that there is no single or right way to confront all the issues and emotions stirred by cancer. We've discovered the widest spectrum of responses and insights during the preparation of this book, from being ignored by family and friends to being suffocated by all the attention. Our mission was to give all parties the tools with which to address everything from neglect to hovering.

Some people will say, *"If they love me, they'll know what to do for me."* We hate to break this bit of news to you, but nobody can read minds, let alone when those thoughts can fluctuate greatly during a cancer crisis. Even couples who have been married a half-century can be confused by what the other is thinking and saying at a time like this. It's human nature.

✎ Read
✎ Listen
✎ Talk

This book was originally designed to be a guidebook for family and friends on how to assist the patient/survivor. During the process, we discovered that survivors sometimes need tips or a dose of encouragement to articulate those needs. Communication is, as they say, a two-way street.

We wanted to find out what did and didn't work for patients/survivors and their family and friends. To explore these thoughts and ideas, we sent out a survey, with the cooperation of the Cancer Center for Healthy Living Inc., to individuals in central Illinois affected by cancer. Within these pages, you will find the responses to questions we posed to them — survivors and their loved ones — seeking their insights, experiences, perceptions and wisdom.

They opened our eyes to a wide range of emotions that are universal and often contradictory. Some were heartbreaking to read, while others lifted our spirits. And we know there are many others out there who can understand what these folks told us. Look for survivor quotes that include their first name, age and type of cancer. Family and friends include their first name, age, relative with cancer and the kind. They're presented as written on the surveys, incomplete sentences and all, because the message is more important than the grammar.

Memo to myself

✎ Fill in the blanks
✎ Tear out and keep
✎ Copy and use again
✎ Share thoughts with loved ones

Don't be intimidated by the size of this book. It's designed to be picked up and tackled or absorbed if you have five minutes or five hours. It's even printed on off-white paper to make it easier on the eyes. It's meant for everyone, though some sections may be targeted to one more than the other. Check out the "Top responses" for a quick overview. Use the memos with the pencils, as shown above, to jot down your own responses and thoughts in a particular section. Please take time to reflect on the words compiled by Robin Unes and her fellow survivors on the *"Just one of many"* pages. Feel free to duplicate the checklists and worksheets if you choose to use them on more than one occasion. Some concepts are covered in more than one section. *We've created this book for you and yours.*

You will notice that throughout, you will see the word "survivor" used more often than "patient" because the focus is on physical and emotional survival, even though we know that every story does not have a happy ending. A section on death and dying was imperative to help people during that most difficult of times, when communication can help ease the pain and grief. However, we do subscribe to Robin's theory that for every day after the diagnosis, everyone is a survivor, no matter how many days or years that is.

We want you to remember the following "secrets" as you go through this volume:

12

▶ *No two people are alike or respond the same way. What works for one may never work for another.*

▶ *You don't need to have a prepared speech to communicate with someone you care about.*

▶ *Some people are afraid to show their emotions because they consider it a sign of weakness. Remember: It's actually a sign of strength to admit you're human.*

Also keep these points in mind:

▶ *Always check with your physician or healthcare provider about any suggestions in this book, i.e., exercise or massage. This is not a medical guide nor does it claim to be.*

▶ *Do not hesitate to consult with a mental health professional to deal with issues such as depression. This book is not a substitute for professional counseling.*

Always remember, as we go through life, we have no idea whose life we have touched. It will amaze you how many people care about and want to assist you, whether you're the survivor or a family member or friend.

We hope we have fulfilled Robin Unes' goal, articulated in her plans for her book …

"This book is written to help those who know someone who is dealing with cancer. The advice comes from actual cancer survivors and their families. Hopefully it will provide some helpful ideas to ease the stress and make it easier to help your friend through the difficult times related to cancer."

'You have cancer'

You're never quite the same after you hear that diagnosis for yourself or for a loved one: *"You have cancer."* There's only one guarantee in that moment: *Your life will change forever.*

No matter the prognosis, treatment or outcome, cancer changes the patient's life and the lives that revolve around them. The bad news? It will be a battle unlike any other. The good news? Survivors, family and friends more often than not take a new approach to life: *They appreciate life and each other more.*

And that's good, very, very good.

The patient/survivor, *should not* and *does not* have to make this journey alone. One of the greatest healing powers in this world is the human connection and its powerful effects on our physical, emotional and spiritual well-being. We can benefit by learning how to communicate effectively with those who love us.

Emotional pain can be as or more taxing than physical pain, and that's why everyone involved must not be afraid to speak up *and* listen. Both actions require courage and even more compassion.

That's why cancer patients must reach out, and family and friends must reach in.

Easier said than done, you say, but not when you have the tools, the words and the willingness to understand. We know that medical expertise works to rid the body of the physical disease, but we also believe that compassion and communication can enhance and heal the body, mind and spirit.

It's time to face the realities … and the possibilities.

"Don't be afraid. Even if you don't know what to say, make contact."
Ann, 45, breast

Ideas of support & comfort to share with someone just diagnosed with cancer

14

Our survivors were very expressive about what they believed would be helpful for those newly diagnosed with cancer. It's important to consider that this is only advice, which was born in a place of introspection and personal experience. These suggestions are *their* priorities and what helped them stay strong, resilient and focused on their recovery.

▶ Keep up a "normal" routine

▶ Cry when you need to cry

▶ Obtain good physicians

▶ Get as much knowledge and information as possible

▶ Talk about your cancer openly

▶ Ask for assistance

▶ Stay active

▶ Maintain a "healthful" living style, including healthy food

▶ Talk to someone who has gone through cancer

▶ View cancer as a blessing, rather than a curse

▶ Pray

▶ Have an attitude that expects success

▶ Be surrounded by a good nursing staff

▶ Obtain knowledge about the cancer, treatment and options

▶ Obtain your children's support and spend more time with them

▶ Know you are not alone

▶ Keep your spirits high

▶ Have friends who listen

▶ Create an oncology health-care team that you can trust

▶ Maintain your personal determination

▶ Have a partner or trusted friend who also attends physician appointments

▶ Identify a patient advocate

▶ Live for each moment and live life to the fullest

▶ Know that you will be heard and listened to vs. being judged for your choices

▶ Utilize a supportive partner or friend

▶ Maintain an exercise program such as walking

- Get plenty of rest
- Reach out for assistance from other survivors
- Attend a support group
- Be grateful
- Keep an open mind
- Put your trust in God
- Be a good example
- Stay positive
- Get a second opinion
- Stay busy "to keep your mind off the problem"
- Surround yourself with family and close friends
- Talk about other things besides the cancer
- Be your own advocate and push for what you need
- Be calm ... don't overreact
- Ask questions to gather understanding
- Discuss the diagnosis and prognosis
- Be aggressive in your treatment
- Look for alternative treatments
- Look for good inspirational material to read

- Realize how much life is worth living
- Be honest about your feelings
- Use humor and read joke books or watch funny movies
- Do what your physician suggests
- Create a symptom note-book that can be reviewed with your oncology team during office visits
- Meditate and do Tai Chi
- Pay attention to any symptoms and discuss with your oncologist
- Get out and do things
- Seek counseling
- Pay attention to your instincts
- Try to believe that miracles do happen

Top responses

- Don't give up
- Stay positive
- Pray
- Have confidence in physician
- Talk openly

Just one of many

16   My cancer journey began at the age of 32. Like my mom and older sister, a positive biopsy revealed breast cancer. Although my microscopic involvement was caught on a screening mammogram, the cancer had already spread to my lymph system. At the time, my three young children were just 1, 3 and 5. The following months were frightening and devastating to my whole circle of friends and family.

     Three years later after a short remission, I was diagnosed with a recurrence throughout my bones. We were once again faced with many challenges that affected everyone close to me.

     Now it has been five years and my disease is considered stable but continues to require ongoing chemotherapy and bone treatments. In addition to my family and my faith, my support has come largely from my friends. Several friends have confided that at times they were at a loss for what to say or do as I went through these difficult times.

     After the initial diagnosis, most everyone gets the feeling of being in shock. Everything seems unsure as many people are faced with the thought of death for the first time. The world seems strange as it continues to act normally when your own life has turned upside down. This onslaught of emotions can interrupt sleep, cause great anxiety and make even the little things in life seem like near impossible tasks. The feeling of being alone and frightened is common, even though many people are surrounded by loved ones.

17

This is a time when friends can make a big difference and help ease the fear and uncertainty. Sending cards, small gifts or calling will mean a lot to your friend. Sometimes the commotion can be overwhelming, but it is much more appreciated than most people would guess. Your friend with cancer will enjoy knowing that others care and are keeping them in their thoughts.

When we find out about a friend's illness, especially cancer, it is often hard to know just what to do. Many friends worry about saying the wrong thing, intruding on family time or being a bother. It's hard to know if your friend will want to talk about it right away, or prefer time to let it sink in. How to approach your friend depends a lot on their personality. If they tend to be fairly private and quiet, they may not want a lot of questions right away. If you are a very close friend, they may desperately need someone to talk to who will just listen and give support and encouragement.

Robin

Survivors say...

Because of your experience, what would you say or do now if someone you know is diagnosed with cancer?

▸ Tell them how hard things would be, but you can get better. *Karen, 51, lung*

▸ Tell them to never give up hope. New treatments are being discovered every day. *B, 93, breast*

▸ Acceptance of the diagnosis and go for the treatment with a very positive attitude. *Noor, 56, breast*

▸ Give that person lots of hugs. *Donna, 72, colon*

▸ Tell them to imagine themselves becoming healthy. *Diane, 47, breast*

▸ Give my sincere support and love. It can be a lonely time. *Elaine, 72, leukemia*

▸ Tell them how sorry I am, how rotten cancer is, but I know they can get through it. *S, 61, breast*

▸ "You are not alone" and mean it! *Diana, 46, lung*

▸ Call and share my experience, both good and bad, so they know it is normal to fear the unknown. *Mary, 64, breast*

▸ Offer my concern, prayers and to do specific jobs. Do washing, transport kids to activities, run sweeper on regular basis. *Judith, 70, breast*

▸ Give them some hope because I'm an example of someone who's made it. Tell them that their attitude is everything. *Karen, 33, breast*

▸ Remind them it is "beatable." Just concentrate on ridding yourself of cancer cells. *Sandy, 58, breast*

▸ Take it one day and step at a time. *Bill, 64, throat and tongue*

▸ I would give them a shoulder to cry on. *Ana, 35, breast*

- Respect their wishes, follow their lead and help with whatever they need. *Paula, 53, uterine and breast*

- Reach out if you need to. Don't keep everything inside. Talk to others, meditate, pray, get counseling if you need to. *Mary Ann, 56, colon*

- I would tell them to read Lance Armstrong's book. *Murray, 64, lymphoma*

- Try to answer questions they have and fears they are experiencing. *Marilyn, 72, breast*

- Phone, (send a) card, (visit) in person. Reassure them that the feelings they are experiencing are normal. Great strides have been made in treating cancer. *Barbara, 48, breast*

- You can survive it and actually become stronger because of it. *Julie, 61, breast*

- Accept your diagnosis. You can then minimize the fear that results. You must own the fear or the fear will own you. Even on your darkest days, do not lose hope. You can survive. *Jennifer, 42, breast*

- Let them know you can beat it! I've told many people that during chemo, (you should) avoid large crowds. Don't get run down during crucial times after treatments (when blood count can drop), and drink lots and lots of water. *Lorraine, 48, breast*

- Help them to focus on what needs to be done now. Each stage from knowledge to surgery needs to be addressed. Don't try to figure it all out. Take it one step at a time. *D, 42, breast*

- Be available, extend an open invitation to talk anytime. Be as optimistic as is realistically possible. *Clair, 55, breast*

"Adversity does teach who your real friends are."
Lois McMaster Bujold

Help loved ones and friends react to diagnosis

Our survivors gave us clues into what they believe are some important suggestions for significant others and friends at the time of diagnosis:

▸ Keep in touch with the survivor

▸ Help your survivor with tasks

▸ Give encouragement that they will recover

▸ Don't give expectations to achieve

▸ Just "be" with your survivor

▸ Help them with yard work and things around the house

▸ Don't offer advice, wait to be asked

▸ Don't be afraid to talk to your loved one … even if you don't know what to say, just make contact

▸ Take the survivor out to lunch or carryout from a favorite restaurant

▸ Help to gather information about the specific cancer

▸ Ask about how your loved one is coping

▸ Offer support and empathy

▸ Help your survivor with transportation

▸ Offer to do errands

▸ Just love them

▸ Don't ask … just do

▸ Make phone calls for your survivor

▸ Offer hope and assurances

▸ Remind the survivor not to give up

▸ Be patient

▸ Create an e-mail tree where updates can be given to extended family and friends

▸ Go with your survivor to chemotherapy

▸ Talk about all the assistance available at the American Cancer Society or a similar cancer support center

▸ Tell your loved one "we can talk anytime day or night"

▸ Give them lots of hugs

▸ Bring over meals

▶ Make sure the survivor knows you love them and care for them

▶ Keep them in your prayers

▶ Let the survivor know they are important

▶ Send cards of encouragement

▶ Help the survivor without asking

▶ Attend support groups with the survivor

▶ Remind them of all the new medical advances

▶ Talk openly about feelings

Top responses

✏ Keep in touch
✏ Pray
✏ Just listen

What can I do?

✏ _____

✏ _____

✏ _____

✏ _____

✏ _____

✏ _____

Survivors say...

What do you do when your loved one is diagnosed with cancer?

▶ First, just listen, let them talk, then ask, "Is there something I could do for you, something you need or want? Or just call and we can talk any time." A hug, and please be patient when I cry or get angry. I need lots of understanding, patience and lots of encouragement. *Alveretta, 85, ovarian*

▶ Talk about it. Don't walk around on tippy toes. A lot of hugs are in order. You need to know you are loved. *Donna, 72, colon*

▶ Support and love the person. My sister's husband ignored her and was always busy at work when she was fighting cancer. *Elaine, 72, leukemia*

▶ Help research, talk about the future. *Tracy, 33, cervical*

▶ Accept it and pray. My friend recently lost her husband. I was there for her and her family. *Dorothy, 70, breast*

▶ Come to them and let them know that you care. By all means, try to treat them naturall, and without denial. *Robert, 70, lung*

▶ Pray about it, then be your same self. Talk positively without constant reference to the patient's limitations. *Rosalie, 80, breast*

▶ Make contact with the relatives of a cancer patient as it means so much to them. They are usually very anxious to talk about it, whether they are a spouse, child, parent or sibling. *Diane, 47, breast*

▶ Be there with a listening ear and a broad shoulder. Go to support groups and learn about what to expect from that day forward in the future. *Diana, 46, lung*

▶ Accept it and carry on a nearly normal life as possible. Encourage healthful living. Encourage the "patient" to remain as active as possible. *Judith, 70, breast*

▶ Sympathize, but treat it matter-of-factly. You're not dead 'til you're dead. Do what the doctors advise. *Betty, 68, breast*

▶ Show you care. No preaching. *Dona, 74, NA*

- They will survive the shock. If you let cancer be a blessing rather than a curse, you will survive and be a better person. *T, 64, breast*

- Give them a short period of time to grasp what is happening, then call to see how they are coping. Ask questions in order to understand and discuss their diagnosis and prognosis. *Mary, 64, breast*

- Tell them how much you love them and remind them medical advances are being made to help them. *John, 81, prostate and colon*

- Hang in there! Listen to their bodies. Ask for assistance if you need or want it. *V, 66, breast*

- Be knowledgeable about the type of cancer. Keep in contact. Help them stay positive, keep active. *Jude, 64, breast*

- Not to be maudlin. Stay upbeat. Be there, but don't hover. Call occasionally. Don't overact or overreact. *Sandy, 58, breast*

- Help take care of the daily things that they won't or shouldn't worry about. Be understanding. They will go through many different emotions. *Karen, 33, breast*

- Provide physical, emotional, nutritional and humorous support for the duration of healing and treatment and recovery, not just post-op. *Judy, 52, breast*

> "There's no substitution for love." Mary, 62, breast

- Tell them what you are feeling or thinking. It gives them permission to hear how you feel, too. Good or bad days, just be there to listen, call without any reason, send a card, and let them know they are in your prayers. Tell them about all the great things at the cancer center. *Paula, 53, uterine and breast*

- Be calm. Just be with them. Make phone calls for them. Let them know that it's not a death sentence. *Bill, 64, throat and tongue*

- Go to doctor's appointments and take notes on what is said. Let the person vent even if irrational. Encourage them to keep a journal. If you see that help is needed, do it. Don't be afraid to cry with them while giving encouragement and hope. *Mary, 52, breast*

- Talk to them all the time whether they respond or not. They need to feel like you care. Send cards often. Visit by phone or in person. Hugs help immensely. Most of us are moms that have always put themselves last. *Bee, 69, breast*

▶ I will never forget the first phone call from one of my dearest friends when she found out. She cried on the phone, and I was very touched by her emotion. *Ann, 45, breast*

▶ Please don't sum up a diagnosis with something you read about a type of cancer, or someone you know with cancer. Everyone's journey is different! *Diane, 38, thyroid*

▶ Ask what they need from you. No false reassurances. Only my doctors were able to reassure me in any meaningful way. Stay in touch. Not every day, but a lot. Send cards and notes. Be sure they don't go to the first chemo alone, too scary with anticipation. *Karen, 62, breast*

▶ Listen. Let them vent. Cry, rage, rant. Find other survivors to talk to your loved one. They could also talk to survivors and families of survivors for insight. *Theresa, 49, breast*

▶ I'm sure each family is different, but to verbalize how I was feeling was very important to me and helped so much. Try to forgive the patient when they are crabby or mean. *Carolyn, 70, colon*

▶ Ask if there is someone to take her small children when she is having surgery. Offer rides to treatment. Bring meals. Just offering makes her feel better, even if she doesn't take you up on the offer. *Martha, 51, breast*

▶ Don't treat them like a leper. No one has all the answers or can understand how you feel, but the cancer patient can let them into their feelings. Just be yourself on both sides. *Nancy, 57, non-Hodgkins lymphoma*

▶ Give them access to knowledge that you might have about their condition without being too outspoken against their decision or doctors. *Julie, 61, breast*

▶ I have one out-of-town friend who has sent me a card every week for two years! I have another who left "surprises" on my porch every month or so for a year! *Helen, 72, lung*

▶ Get all the knowledge possible, but not go overboard. It's okay to be mad, angry, to cry, yet don't quit living, enjoying life or lose your laughter. *Sara, 35, lung*

▶ I have friends in Minneapolis and Springfield going through chemo and radiation. I e-mail them to try to be their cheerleader. We celebrate the end of chemo, the growth of hair, the end of radiation. We discuss being ill and compare notes. I try to suggest simple comfort ideas that helped me. *Jeannie, 60, breast*

24

My reaction

When someone is diagnosed with cancer, the emotions of every-one involved tend to span the spectrum. The emotions you feel may be uncomfortable. Perhaps you will feel helpless or hopeless. Some loved ones say they feel angry or guilty. In an effort to "normalize" your feelings, we've included the emotions that our caregivers experienced when learning about the diagnosis. Please remember that your feelings can change many times throughout your journey. No one emotion is true for everyone, nor is one emotion constant throughout the time span. Note your responses on these two pages.

Disbelief _____

Anger _____

Numb _____

Overwhelmed _____

Sad _____

Fearful _____

Helpless _____

Dread _____

Unsettled _____

Concerned _____

Uncertain _____

Scared _____

Shocked _____

Determined _____

Love _____

over

Cancer: Here's how YOU can help ME cope & survive

Hopeful _____

Denial _____

Guilt _____

Depressed _____

Unfairness _____

Worried _____

Rage _____

Upset _____

Devastated _____

Regret _____

Horror _____

Frustration _____

Hopeless _____

Not surprised _____

Panic _____

Confusion _____

Out of control _____

Acceptance _____

Hurt _____

Resentment _____

Compassion _____

Anxiety _____

Sorrow _____

Annoyed _____

Courageous _____

Cancer proves to be an abrupt wake-up call

Cancer has a way of changing a person's priorities. Diane Cullinan Oberhelman learned that the hard way at age 36.

This central Illinois commercial developer remembers the daily routine before an aggressive case of breast cancer slammed on the brakes in every facet of her life in 1995.

"I was very driven, but with different goals and priorities than I have now. A lot of the smaller problems bothered me more. I wasn't as focused on my personal relationships with the exception of my four children (then ages 8-16)," says this woman who exudes more energy than many women half her age.

A rainy July the Fourth in 1995 gave Diane more of a jolt than the fireworks that graced American skies that night.

Lesson #1
Don't wait for cancer to determine your life's priorities

"I was taking the day off with the kids, and we were playing hide and go seek. I was hiding behind one of the beds. We were hot, sweaty. I scratched on my right side, not quite under my arm, but I felt this huge lump. I thought, 'What in the world was that?' I felt it again. I had never felt that before. I felt my left side and there wasn't one there. 'This isn't right. This is a bad sign.' "

She had ignored her mother's earlier advice. "My mom had been saying, 'Diane, I know they say 40 years old for mammograms, but you should go in now for a baseline. It would be a good idea.' "

She immediately called her (then) sister-in-law, Dr. Theresa Falcon, a gynecologist, and asked her to check it. The doctor said it was highly unlikely it was anything serious because of her age, but recommended that she get it examined further. Diane didn't want to concern her family, so she saw a physician who performed a needle biopsy on a Friday. While waiting for the results, she had a nagging ache that something was not right.

Though she remained generally optimistic, "A sixth sense told me that something terrible was wrong." There had been no history of cancer in the family.

"I can still picture this doctor. He scooted up on his little brown chair, took my hand, and said, 'I have bad news.' That was quite traumatic, and I was all by my myself." She broke the news to her then-husband and waited. She convinced herself that it would require only a lumpectomy, a blip on the radar screen of life.

She then told her four children, "Mom has something to tell you," an approach she soon regretted because that set the stage for immediate panic for a long time afterward if she started any conversation with those same scary words. However, she explained it was "a small operation, a small cancer." She says kids know when you're trying to gloss something over. If she had to do it again, she would have been more honest with them and told them it was more serious and outlined her "game plan." Being too upbeat and positive can be counterproductive, she says with the benefit of hindsight.

Upon further testing, it was discovered to be an aggressive cancer. She didn't research options. Her oncologist and then-brother-in-law, Dr. Stephen Cullinan, recommended a mastectomy; the surgeon suggested a lumpectomy. She now believes it is better to have the oncologist as the primary and surgeon as the secondary. She believes being aggressive saved her life.

Confronting a major challenge at work, Diane didn't let on what was happening to her personally. She foolishly postponed her surgery, admitting now that she obviously did not have her priorities in order, because she was more worried about business than her own life. She was more focused on the individuals she worked with and how her cancer could affect their lives.

However, a scan showed that the cancer had gone into her lymph nodes. She was devastated, her hopes dashed for an "in and out." She said, "I'll do whatever it takes, every single item on the menu, to get rid of this." The mastectomy in August 1995 alone was not going to do the job.

A stem cell transplant was highly recommended. Then she learned that more than 20 percent of the patients at that time died, not from the cancer, but from the procedure. She was determined to be a survivor. But she was still the same old CEO Diane, worried about what she wouldn't be able to do. She resisted cutting back and accepting that she couldn't do everything.

Now she finds it hard to believe that she didn't put aside work

> **Lesson #2**
> Don't go to the doctor by yourself

28

even as she came to grips with what was most important in life ... life itself. Her parents and doctors encouraged the most aggressive treatment, and her children were supportive, yet devastated, though they tried to be positive.

Diane kept up her own positive persona, though now she believes she should have talked about the negatives and confronted them at the time. Despite her generally positive attitude, she knew it was not realistic. Emptiness swept her. Her friends and co-workers were wonderful and would have done anything for her if she had asked. Yet again, she still didn't have her priorities in order. She foolishly scheduled chemotherapy treatments at 3 p.m. Fridays so she'd be sick on the weekends and be able to go back to work on Monday. She realizes she should have given her family that time. She shakes her head.

"Shame on me!"

She also acknowledges that those who surrounded her told her what she wanted to hear and were positive, though she could sense they were extremely worried. She needed to take control of the cancer by shaving her head before all of her hair fell out. Then she proudly went to work bald for the annual Halloween party as Mr. Clean. When she did wear a wig, sometimes she'd pull it off to make others laugh.

Lesson #3
Admit you can't do everything and that people are very willing to help you

Her sister, Laura, served as donor for platelets, which hadn't improved after an autologous stem cell transplant in Iowa City in mid-October. She had originally scheduled the surgery for November — again to accommodate her work schedule better — but the transplant was moved up because of an opening and her urgent status. She couldn't imagine being gone for a month and vowed to work while in the hospital. She promised her kids and everybody "three weeks max."

"I felt like I had let people down. Somehow it was my fault I had cancer. I felt so badly for my family, my co-workers, my friends. It aged my parents. They had 12-hour shifts for two months because I was so sick. They nursed me back to health."

Her saddest thoughts were of her parents as she observed them watching her. Now she felt like a huge burden. This went on for two and a half months, existing in a sterile environment. Feeling like something out of a monster movie, she looked so different that she was sure the kids were embarrassed during their Sunday visits. Silently, she was so sick, discouraged and desperate.

However, due to her weakened immune system, Diane was literally in for the fight of her life as fungal pneumonia nearly killed her. It was in her left lung, and she fought a fever of 105 degrees with medication and covered with ice packs. She flew home for Christmas Eve but succumbed to fever again and was immediately flown back to Iowa City in the middle of the night. By then she comprehended how vulnerable, helpless and dangerously close to death she was.

Diane also learned much about herself as she learned to take care of herself again, including toting around a machine protecting her with an antibiotic drip. For a long time, she had around-the-clock nursing care, and missed so much being home and part of everyday activities.

Though she just didn't believe it herself at the time, now she tells patients/survivors that others *do* want to help them. Through the years, she's discovered an amazing number of cancer patients who refuse to ask for help because they're afraid of becoming a burden.

Many of the women she knew during her treatment didn't make it, and she's seen the effect on their children, the void the loss of that person leaves in their lives. She encourages all patients to fight as these women had. "It's a battle worth fighting. You're hurting your families if you don't fight."

She never considered not fighting. That's just who she is. She fought for the sake of her family, because she knew it would be more devastating if she were not here. There is no greater love than unconditional love for family. "You're expected to do everything you can to survive for each other."

She admires the strength of her children and their enthusiasm and energy in helping start a Peoria branch of Komen Kids, which evolved into Kids Konnected. She's extremely proud of them and knew that the experience would help them and other families. Cancer can and should bring a family closer together, though it is one of the most difficult ordeals a family can face.

Getting back into the real world proved to be difficult, challenging and sometimes felt impossible. However, she views this new world much differently and appreciates life much more. She remarried and spends much more time with loved ones and friends. She wants cancer patients and their loved ones and friends to be able to communicate, to be more comfortable with each other.

"I think it was a blessing that it was a more serious cancer, because it changed my life for the better. I reprioritized."

Lesson #4

Cancer can be a blessing instead of a curse

My priorities

Rank them with #1 as most important

Rating MY priorities BEFORE cancer

____Career

____Family

____Friendships

____Hobbies

____Material possessions

____Money

____Professional achievements

____Social status

____Other _____

____Other _____

____Myself as a whole

____My physical health

____My emotional health

____Spouse/significant other

____Children

____Parents

____Faith

Rating MY priorities AFTER cancer

____Career

____Family

____Friendships

____Hobbies

____Material possessions

____Money

____Professional achievements

____Social status

____Other _____

____Other _____

____Myself as a whole

____My physical health

____My emotional health

____Spouse/significant other

____Children

____Parents

____Faith

"Be there & listen to their spouse's needs."
Ana, 35, breast

over

What was the biggest change? _____

Why? _____

_____

_____

_____

What changed the least? _____

Why? _____

_____

_____

_____

What should have changed but didn't? _____

Why? _____

_____

_____

_____

What do I want to change? _____

Why? _____

_____

_____

How will I do it? _____

_____

_____

_____

_____

When? _____

"Hold on. It's a rough ride. Pray a lot." Carol, 71, colon

Loved ones say...

Their reactions to hearing of a loved one's cancer and how that affected their feelings toward that person.

Harsh realities & anger

▸ Hurt, anger, yet not surprised. He smoked 40-plus years. *Georgia, 48, father, lung*

▸ Disbelief, numb, then anger. My dad is *so* healthy. He does everything he's supposed to, eats right, exercises tons, is in incredible physical shape. It kills me to see him have to go through this and the worst is yet to come! *Laura, 44, father, prostate*

▸ Devastation, especially after I found out that my sister knew something was seriously wrong but did nothing. *Rosemary, 66, sister, ovarian*

▸ I knew it was a matter of time. She knew it, too. She cut filters off her cigarettes. Started smoking at about 15. *Len, 51, sister, lung*

▸ Anger. I knew he had been ill for months, and I couldn't get him to go to the doctor. *Linda, 62, husband, colon*

▸ Extreme sadness, depression, denial, hopelessness. I was pregnant, and we had a 2-year-old son. This wasn't supposed to happen. Why does God have to take away someone when you really love each other, but couples that hate each other get to stay together for 20-30-50 years? *Monica, 35, husband, pancreatic*

▸ Shocked! How can this be happening again? *Fred, 63, wife, breast*

▸ I had to discuss what this illness would mean to us and our young family. *Bette, 57, husband, melanoma*

▸ I was shocked and confused. Mom was always going to the doctor for other reasons. How could they have missed the cancer? *Rue, 29, mother, breast*

Determination & optimism

▸ Feeling the need to get going, take care of the problem and get back to normal. *Darrell, 54, wife, lung*

▶ Fear, concern, a desire to be supportive and "there" for him. *Judith, 70, husband, colon*

▶ I was married three months to my high school sweetheart. I was as determined as he was to get him healthy again so we could enjoy our marriage. *Marianne, 71, husband, large cell lymphoma*

▶ My dad was diagnosed and died when he was 75. My first reaction was great sadness, but also a determination to enjoy him. *Mary, 42, father, lung*

▶ I felt a sense of urgency to get through this crisis and have her health restored ASAP, but I remember thinking, "just be support-ive and positive because this is going to be a journey back to health and wellness. Move forward in faith, not fear." *Lori, 39, partner, breast*

▶ I am a nurse with former oncology experience, and I was the one who discovered the lump in his neck. With the knowledge I had, I was preparing for the worse, yet tried to be hopeful it wasn't cancer. *Mary, 48, husband, thyroid*

> "We have to fight this together."
> Doug, 57, wife, breast

▶ Sadness, too young, too vibrant, too caring. If anyone could "lick" this disease, he could. *Roger, 56, and Char, 59, friend, prostate*

Helplessness & fear

▶ Fear. She doesn't follow-up. *Jean, 64, mother, cervical*

▶ Like the sky was falling. Like my life as I knew it was over. Inability to think or breathe correctly for a while. *Liz, 43, sister, breast*

▶ She didn't deserve this, sad. She was a loving, good person, unconditional friend, generous. *P, 66, sister-in-law, lung and bone*

▶ Fear, anxiety, gut-wrenching sorrow. *Vera, 73, several relatives with cancer*

▶ Fearful. Always my mother was strong, never really sick, the strength of her family. I knew she would not complain or let her children know how she suffered as she became weaker. *L, 50, mother, lung*

▶ Because I didn't know what it was, I wasn't afraid. Dad had out-lived all his friends. and he was never emotional, so I wasn't. *Abbie, 51, father, leukemia*

▸ I was afraid of losing her. I felt helpless because I couldn't do anything to make the cancer go away. *Bill, 59, wife, breast*

▸ I responded by mowing his lawn. I was afraid I was going to break down crying. I didn't want him to see that because I was afraid it would frighten him. After all, he was still alive. *Jeanne, 53, father, liver*

▸ Total devastation. She was my only daughter, my best friend and the love of my life. *Annamarie, 62, daughter, NA*

▸ Worried that she might die. *Dan, 44, wife, breast*

▸ We couldn't believe it. She had a mammogram every year. Radiologists went back and checked previous x-rays. Could not believe it had progressed to lymph nodes. *Ralph, 68, wife, breast*

▸ Fear, hope, disbelief. We were the same age. Why her, not me? *Diane, 38, friend/co-worker, breast*

▸ Cheated out of our friendship. Scared the treatments would kill her. *Susan, 49, best friend, lymphoma*

▸ How I wished I could have taken her place so she would not have to suffer. My mother never smoked. My dad always did but quit 10 years ago after his father did. I wish my husband would quit. *L, 50, mother, lung*

"*Horror, fear, a deep feeling of love.*" Bertha, 84, husband, prostate

▸ Very sad. My friend and I (both nurses) had the feeling that she would not survive. *Sharon, 65, friend, breast*

▸ First fear, then hope that it was caught early enough. *David, 67, wife, breast*

▸ Fear of the unknown, shock, the stigma of cancer, but really took it fairly well in stride. *Paul, 53, wife, breast*

▸ Sheer terror and shock. She had never been sick nor been in a hospital since the birth of her children (except for hernia repair). *Nancy, 67, mother, pancreatic*

▸ Initially numb, then immediately scared. *Jean, 64, mother, cervical*

▸ Shock, wondered how my mother would handle the news. *Julie, 51, father, lung*

▸ I was mostly scared and unsure of what might happen. Also, I was at an age when I wanted everything to be normal, status quo. I felt annoyed, angry, etc., that this happened to my family. *Maureen, 23, mother, breast*

▶ It was very difficult to see my parents so blown away by the diagnosis. I wanted to be near both of them. *Carlene, 51, mother, breast*

▶ I am afraid that I didn't say anything. I just did what I could to be of help to Mom while Dad was gone to the doctor or hospital. *Abbie, 51, father, leukemia*

By their side

▶ My father, younger sister and I were with her July 2, 2000, when the doctors found a tumor in the lung, bronchial tube, and it could be removed with an operation. I gave her a box of chocolates and said life is like a box of chocolates, you never know what you're going to get. *L, 50, mother, lung*

▶ I was with him during the time he was given the diagnosis, and I'd prepared him also for the potential that this was cancer. We had our fears confirmed and knew that he needed surgery and treatment to beat this. *Mary, 48, husband, thyroid*

▶ We were together when the diagnosis was made. We cried, we hugged, we asked why and how. I reassured her that we were in this together. *Mark, 45, wife, breast*

▶ I couldn't let my feelings or emotions enter into it. I was in the doctor's office with my parents. Originally we were told it was a 1 percent chance of cancer. I had to begin taking notes immediately. *Carlene, 51, mother, breast*

▶ Speechless, as I was there when she was told the news over the phone. *Sandi, 51, sister, ovarian*

A brave face

▶ I tried to conceal most of my concerns, fears. *Wayne, 48, wife, breast*

▶ I tried to be brave. I broke down when I saw my brother in the hall after seeing my mother. *Lois, 53, mother, breast*

▶ I tried to express feelings of hope in spite of the diagnosis. *Rosemary, 66, sister, ovarian*

▶ I tried to be calm, comforting, optimistic and tried very hard to hide the tears. *Bertha, 84, husband, prostate*

▶ Always felt we would be together no matter what. *Robert, 53, wife, breast and uterine*

▶ Tried to be as supportive as possible. Also cried a lot in private. *Rose, 70, husband, lymphoma*

▶ My job was not to react or respond, but to be available for input, an outlet for her feelings and desires. *Leonard, 41, wife, breast*

▶ Never tried to let the fear show outside myself. *L, fiancee, kidney*

▶ Cried, tried to joke about baldness, assured her we would get her through it. *Monica, 52, sister, NA*

Inspired by them

▶ I couldn't believe how brave she was and the positive attitude she had. *Bill, 59, wife, breast*

▶ Positive reinforcement, "we'll deal with it and move on." *John, 55, wife, breast*

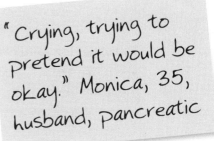

" Crying, trying to pretend it would be okay." Monica, 35, husband, pancreatic

▶ She was so incredibly positive, I was so comfortable just hanging out. *Laura, 44, aunt, lymph*

▶ Her strength gave me strength. I realized I had to be there for her because she was so determined to conquer the lymphoma. *Susan, 49, best friend, lymphoma*

▶ With faith, determination and love. *Patricia, 64, husband, larynx*

▶ Positive. Let's do as the doctor tells us, see what the test results are, take each day as it comes. *Georgia, 48, father, lung*

▶ Kept our relationship the same. Didn't want to play the "poor me" role. Hoped that faith, love and determination would make a difference. *Mary, 42, father, lung*

▶ Told her that she would not have to deal with this alone. *Bernard, 80, wife, breast*

▶ Admiration for her determination to get back to normal. On the tennis court three weeks after surgery. *Lois, 53, mother, breast*

▶ Love and admiration for her acceptance of the diagnosis. Mother had a calming effect on me. *Kay, 65, mother, leukemia*

▶ Proud of her determination. *Chuck, 61, wife, rectal*

▶ Initially no effect, but over time I was amazed by the strength of her spirit. As her disease got worse with the recurrence, she seemed driven to do more for others. *Chris, 38, mother, breast*

▶ More love and admiration as she was not bitter about the mis-diagnosis. *Pam, friend, breast and lung*

A tighter bond

▸ We had that old reality check that "life is short" and you need to be mindful that each day is a gift. *Mary, 48, husband, thyroid*

▸ I certainly didn't love my wife any less. I knew she was going to need me. *Randy, 46, wife, breast*

▸ More love and the feeling I had to provide positive support. *Gerald, 67, wife, breast*

▸ I felt protective of Mom. Like the tables had been switched. I loved her more every day for her courage. *Rue, 29, mother, breast*

▸ I loved him even more and couldn't imagine life without him. *Colleen, 60, husband, colon*

▸ Visited and told him I loved him more often. *Julie, 51, father, lung*

▸ Even when I was scared, I told him every day that I loved him and he could count on me no matter what. *L, fiancee, kidney*

▸ Desired to get closer to her before I lose her. Expressing my feelings and concerns and deep friendship with her. Allowing her to express her needs and feelings. *Kathleen, 49, friend, breast*

▸ He was more verbal about his wishes, but I didn't change my attitude. I learned to like him more. *Abbie, 51, father, leukemia*

▸ Made me realize how much I loved him, stopped taking him for granted or getting mad about small stuff. We grew much closer throughout his illness. *Monica, 35, husband, pancreatic*

▸ I think we became more open and closer. It was to be our fight. *David, 67, wife, breast*

▸ Deeper love, desire to be there for him, to care for him, to "hold on" to him. We were never a physically demonstrative family, but I just wanted to hold his hand and hug him. *Shirley, 66, brother, lung*

▸ We have always been very close, but breast cancer made us closer. Breast cancer made me aware of how much I loved and needed my wife. *Bill, 59, wife, breast*

▸ Wishing she could be with us longer. Being thankful for the time we had together. Knew bone cancer was hard to beat. *P, 66, sister-in-law, lung and bone*

▸ I couldn't love my mom any more than I already did, but I knew she would need a lot of encouragement to move forward. *Carlene, 51, mother, breast*

▶ We have the kind of friendship where we feel we have known each other forever and love each other no matter what. So I could only love her more. I still strive to have the patience and courage she exhibited. *Susan, 49, best friend, lymphoma*

▶ More appreciation, pity. *John, 55, wife, breast*

▶ More love, appreciation for each day alive, realizing we're all mortal. It could just have easily been me. In later stages, while we were close, I developed my own identity as a caregiver. *Paul, 53, wife, breast*

▶ A more gentle feeling, one of caring and wanting to help in anything I could. *Marianne, 71, husband, large cell lymphoma*

▶ More protective, heavier feeling of being responsible for her. *Martha, 50, mother, non-Hodgkins lymphoma*

▶ I realized how much she meant to me and how strong our partnership was. *John, 69, wife, breast*

▶ We became even closer than we already were. We appreciated each other more, looked out for each other more, and "wasted" far less time. *Mark, 45, wife, breast*

▶ Deeper concern, more love. I never wanted him to feel I thought he was going to die. *Lynn, 64, brother, colon*

▶ Wanted to protect him as much as possible. Would have preferred to "do it myself." *Rose, 70, husband, lymphoma*

▶ Protective, more forgiving and loving. More patient with any personal idiosyncrasies. *Sharon, 65, friend, breast*

▶ More love, total fear knowing what she was facing, anger, rage toward God, totally dedicated to taking care of her. *Annamarie, 62, daughter, NA*

▶ More love, always fear. At 82, she was not "old," but a vital, take charge person. *Nancy, 67, mother, pancreatic*

Trying to comprehend

▶ As a listener, then responding to the rest of my family's needs. *James, 55, mother, colon*

▶ Curious about treatment. Asked questions. *A, 25, friend, breast*

▶ I was scared to talk to my mom because I didn't want to act like I wasn't taking this situation seriously, and I didn't know what to say if I were to talk about cancer. *Maureen, 23, mother, breast*

▶ On her initial diagnosis, I did not comprehend the magnitude. I was also living overseas so my coping mechanism was to ignore/deny the situation. I wish I could have understood the magnitude of the situation. *Chris, 38, mother, breast*

▶ Supportive and just let her take the lead until I felt comfortable enough to ask questions. *Rue, 29, mother, breast*

A whirlwind of emotions

▶ I am sure I cried. She had beautiful thick hair and at the prospect of chemo, I immediately had a formal portrait made of both her and my father. *Nancy, 67, mother, pancreatic*

▶ Disbelief, find a way to beat it. Thought we would have had more time together; married less than two years when he died. *Mary, 52, husband, kidney*

▶ Teary-eyed but on the upside. *Donald, 70, wife, lymphoma*

▶ Too numb to really feel. *Carol, 66, mother, breast*

▶ Just let things take their course. "Being there" mostly, listening, assuring that the patient still has *own* identity in spite of being a "cancer patient." *Ann, 51, friend, brain*

▶ Cautious. My dad isn't real open with his emotions, and as a nurse, I "know too much." *Laura, 44, father, prostate*

▶ I tried to be honest. If she was down, I asked if she felt tired or ill. I tried to be honest, not always, "You look great," which many people do. *Diane, 38, friend/co-worker, breast*

▶ I did not think it was right for her to suffer emotionally because she always took good care of herself. *Ron, 62, wife, breast*

▶ I talk about it when he feels like it, but I'm not afraid to talk about it. My mom talks about it so much because she has a need to, but I know he gets sick of it. He just wants the treatment to be over with. *Laura, 44, father, prostate*

▶ It made me appreciate more what I do have. *Dan, 44, wife, breast*

▶ She was capable of making her decisions. I was a sounding board and supported her decisions. *N, 68, friend, breast*

▶ Sometimes fear of saying the wrong thing, or not having anything to say. Silence can be scary. *Diane, 38, friend/co-worker, breast*

▶ Compassion, some fear of outcome, and the fear that I would not be strong enough for her. *Sandi, 51, sister, ovarian*

How to recover from all the losses cancer brings

"We are not powerless specks of dust drifting around in the wind, blown by random destiny. We are, each of us, like beautiful snowflakes — unique, and born for a specific reason and purpose." Elizabeth Kubler-Ross

Cancer represents losses, loss of control, loss of health and more, not just possible death. Loss affects us in many ways, some of which are unexpected. Noted for her expertise in grief and loss, eminent psychiatrist Elizabeth Kubler-Ross has identified five commonly experienced stages of grief and mourning of these various losses.

▸ *Shock and denial.* The first stage includes the temporary shock reflex to the cancer diagnosis. During this time, the survivor, family and loved ones tend to isolate and feel overwhelmed, numb and withdrawn. It is also common for people to avoid the cancer survivor during this initial stage.

▸ *Anger.* During the anger stage the survivor, family and loved ones may be mad at God, or feel angry with people around them. Sometimes the anger at others includes jealousy that others can go on with their life without the invasion of cancer. Anger is sometimes directed at healthcare workers, physicians and hospitals.

▸ *Bargaining.* During the bargaining stage, the survivor or loved ones attempt to bargain with God, their Higher Power, or the Universe. In this stage people tend to promise change, living a more authentic loving existence, being more accepting, or numerous other socially valued behaviors in exchange for health and recovery.

▸ *Depression.* During this stage, the effected have feelings of sadness, tearfulness, disturbed sleep, excessive crying, and sometimes even thoughts of suicide. There is a loss

"I wanted to give her enough space for her to deal with it her way."
Michael, 50, wife

related to current situations (loss of mobility, loss of body parts, loss of relational issues, etc.), as well as preparatory depression related to losses yet to come in the future.

42

▶ *Acceptance.* During this final stage, the survivors and loved ones begin to look for the lessons of the experience. During acceptance, humans tend to focus on hope, resiliency and the powerful act of survivorship. In some cases, the acceptance stage is focusing on the impending death of a loved one, and opening their hearts to allowing final days filled with dignity and love.

"I did not know what to say. You ask questions like, 'Should I carry on with the menial everyday conversation or should we only talk about the diagnosis." Maureen, 23, mother, breast

As many critics of Kubler-Ross have noted, not everyone goes through these stages in the same identical order. In fact some people go in and out of stages on multiple occasions, i.e. you can find yourself feeling depressed during the initial diagnosis and once again during treatment. Some who experience loss and grief may not go through some stages, but most commonly, these are universal icons for the grieving process.

What losses am I feeling?

Denial tough to address

I can't have cancer. I can't be facing surgery. My loved one can't have cancer. The diagnosis is wrong. We'll just ignore this. It can't happen to us, me, our family.

43

Denial is one of the five steps of grieving and loss mostly commonly associated with the diagnosis of a life-threatening illness such as cancer. *(See the steps of grieving any type of loss on page 41.)* This is a natural response in addressing any loss, and not just death. Some patients/survivors refuse to get medical help or continue treatment because of denial, or they may simply "give up," thinking it's fruitless to even fight cancer, and the results can be devastating. Loved ones can deny the impending death of someone stricken by cancer until the final days ... *I didn't believe he/she could die.*

That's the ugly side of cancer: denial, wishful thinking, lost hours and days avoiding reality, time that could have been spent creating priceless opportunities to talk, share and love.

If someone you love is in denial, remember that you can't force them to change their attitude, but you can be consistent and supportive when reality does shatter them. Broad statements don't always soak in. Sometimes people have to hear the direct brutal facts again and again: *"I'm dying ..."* *"You're going to die if you don't start treatment now ..."* Some people may think that's cruel, but perhaps it's crueler if they claim later, *"I didn't know or understand what a difference it would make."*

"She wouldn't let you say the big "c" word. Denial on her part." Virginia, 66, several relatives

Honesty allows the natural process of grieving to begin no matter the individual, the circumstance, the prognosis, the relationship.

▶ Denial. Could not believe it was true. My wife was too healthy. *Tom, 44, wife, breast*

▶ Hard to believe this was happening. I pulled back and isolated. *Bette, 57, husband, melanoma*

▶ My parents kept from the family that some of the cancer had spread to his lymph nodes and that he was given a time frame of five years to live. *Krista, 39, father, prostate*

My reaction

44 Survivor or loved one:
Breaking *the* news, hearing *the* news

What did I say? _____

_____

_____

_____

What did I hear? _____

_____

_____

_____

_____

What do I wish I had said? _____

_____

_____

_____

What do I wish I had heard? _____

_____

_____

_____

Loved ones say...

Did the patient/survivor try to ease your fears about the diagnosis? If so, how specifically, and did this help?

Yes

▶ It felt like I was more upset and scared than she was. I know she was scared, but she was trying to reassure me more than herself. *Barb, 44, best friend, non-Hodgkins lymphoma*

▶ Yes, empathized, considered my feelings. Lived her faith, no matter the outcome, it was okay. *Doug, 57, wife, breast*

▶ He never was fearful or frantic about it. He accepted it and went on to live and carry on as normal as possible. *Judith, 70, husband, colon*

▶ She remained optimistic that she would recover. It didn't help. *John, 55, wife, breast*

▶ He told me everything would be okay, regardless of outcome, gave some comfort. *Bette, 57, husband, melanoma*

▶ Yes, she said she would be fine and "no one lives forever." *Martha, 50, mother, non-Hodgkins lymphoma*

▶ He told me he loved me and would not be able to go through the situation without me. We had hope. *L, fiancee, kidney*

▶ I knew he had been through this two times before. We knew together we would be fine. *Marianne, 71, husband, large cell lymphoma*

▶ My dad had a great sense of humor and often used it! *Mary, 42, father, lung*

▶ Tried to convince herself and me it would be fine. *Len, 51, sister, lung*

▶ Yes, she would not always tell me everything the doctor said and going to do next so I wouldn't worry. *L, 50, mother, lung*

▶ With humor and knowledge. *Ann, 51, friend, brain*

▶ She accepted her diagnosis and counseled others with breast cancer. *Ron, 62, wife, breast*

- She had a very positive attitude, which was contagious. *Gerald, 67, wife, breast*

- My mom is strong in faith and God's power. She's encouraging me. *Bambi, 47, mother and sister, breast*

- He was so positive about the outlook. Unfortunately, we knew too much. *Roger, 56, and Char, 59, friend, prostate*

- We both had a lot to learn. *Robert, 53, wife, breast and uterine*

- Yes, she was always upbeat. Yes, it did help. *Hiles, 69 wife, uterine*

- She said she would be a "cancer conqueror," not just a survivor and definitely not a victim by educating herself and implementing the appropriate "plan of attack," utilizing a blend of holistic and traditional medical modalities and organizing an entire army of health care practitioners, family and friends. *Lori, 39, partner, breast*

- She used humor to explain her latest ills. Often after being with her, you would stop and think, "this is a major change." Things are getting to the end. *Mary, 63, best friend, breast*

- She talked a lot about joining her mom and sister in heaven. She had a lot of peace, which helped others feel peace. *Diane, 38, friend/co-worker, breast*

- He would tell me, "It's going to be all right" or "It could have been worse." This kind of cancer is very treatable. *Mary, 48, husband, thyroid*

- Yes, she would tell me she would win this battle. Before recurrence, yes. After recurrence, we both knew it was a matter of time. *Mark, 45, wife, breast*

- Yes! A lot! It helped but it also made me mad that she didn't act scared. Now I know she couldn't have done it any other way. It helped that we believed her. *Kathleen, 24, mother, breast*

- By telling us she would be all right, my mom was very convincing. It took my grandma at times to "wake" us kids up so we could see the seriousness of the cancer. *Maureen, 23, mother, breast*

No

- No, he knows I know too much as it is. *Laura, 44, father, prostate*

- No, he was depressed. *Patricia, 64, husband, larynx*

- No, he did not talk about it with me. *Julie, 51, father, lung*

- No, but she tried to keep the worst information from me, so I went to her appointments to listen and ask questions. *Rue, 29, mother, breast*

- No, I'm more the optimist and he's the pessimist. *Patti, 52, husband, renal cell cancer*

- Initial diagnosis was not as "life changing" as second time. We were both somewhat in denial at first. *Barbara, 66, husband, larynx*

- No, he wouldn't discuss it and refused to answer questions. It was very hard to anticipate what was needed. *Bertha, 84, husband, prostate*

- Not so much. We didn't talk much about his fears. He hoped the medications would work. *Lynn, 64, brother, colon*

- He was crying but said he wasn't afraid to die. This didn't help me any. *Monica, 35, husband, pancreatic*

> "She was frightened and I knew she was aware of the seriousness of her condition."
> Rosemary, 66, sister, ovarian

Facing facts

- We did not talk of imminent death. *Pat, 57, husband, brain*

- We knew so little about breast cancer that I didn't have enough knowledge to do that. I just let Mom know that I was afraid also. *Carlene, 51, mother, breast*

- We talk facts. *Fred, 63, wife, breast*

- The other way around. I tried to ease her fears by trying to be upbeat and being there for her at any given time. *Leonard, 41, wife, breast*

- Tried to be reassuring. But I gradually grew more and more anxious, fearful and withdrawn, not able to share these with my wife. I had no support system of my own to verbalize my fears. *Paul, 53, wife, breast*

- We both shared the same fears, but also the same confidence. *David, 67, wife, breast*

Talking to your doctor

Do you find yourself clamming up when you are in your doctor's office? Do you feel intimidated? Do they do all the talking and you do all the listening? Do you feel like they are talking to you in some type of foreign language? Are you feeling ill-prepared for the appointment?

Here are some suggestions to make your doctor's appointments a little more comfortable and user-friendly for survivors and loved ones:

▶ *Be prepared by writing down your questions.* Bring paper and pencil to take notes during your appointment. If you feel more comfortable just listening, bring a tape recorder, with the physician's knowledge, to help you keep track of important information, or as a means of explaining things to loved ones. This will also be useful to share with another physician when seeking a second opinion.

▶ *Bring a support person with you (if appropriate) to help you remember important facts or information.* Additionally, your support person can ask questions that you might forget to ask, or help clarify items that were discussed.

▶ *Ask your doctor how much time he has allotted for your visit.* This will help you know how to prioritize your questions. If you don't feel like you've had all of your questions answered, ask how you can arrange additional time to discuss your concerns.

▶ *Talk openly about all of your symptoms and speak up about your concerns.* Be honest about your emotional status, your fears and concerns. Don't leave out any symptoms you've noticed.

▶ *If you feel overwhelmed ... ask your doctor to slow down or repeat what was said in a different way so you can understand more fully.* Don't be embarrassed about asking questions ... your physician is used to answering questions.

▶ *Take a deep breath and ask your physician to wait a minute if you've been given some "difficult" information about your prognosis, diagnosis or treatment options.* Remember, when you are in shock, your body has a natural way of shutting down to protect itself. When your body does that, you won't remember a single thing that your physician has told you during your meeting.

▸ *Bring a list of all of your current medications and always ask about side effects with new medications that are prescribed.* Ask about generic alternatives to save money (but be sure your insurance will cover generic options). Ask your doctor if you can access samples of your medications. Be sure and check with your pharmacist or physician before taking any over-the-counter medicines.

49

▸ *Discuss medical and alternative treatment options.* Ask what had worked for other survivors. Ask about the pros and cons of each. Check into whether you might be eligible for clinical trials. Discuss what they are, if they're safe, their effectiveness, and if insurance will cover them.

▸ *Keep a detailed log of your unusual symptoms, pain, fatigue and stressors that may effect your treatment.* Some cancer survivors find it helpful to keep a food log if they find themselves having adverse reactions to some medications.

▸ *Be sure you ask about the risks and side effects of any and all new medications, treatment procedures, or tests.* It's better to have knowledge vs. being taken by surprise if you didn't ask.

▸ *If you have issues that were not discussed ... make sure you raise the questions yourself.* Too often survivors forget to ask about side effects, complications, degree of effectiveness of the treatment, and prognosis. For patients in their reproductive years, male or female, discuss how your fertility may be affected.

▸ *Ignore your urge to be a "good patient."* More importantly, be an informed and honest patient who advocates for yourself or your loved one. Stay honest and willing to look for options.

▸ *Remember to be assertive, rather than aggressive or passive.* Remember, it is your responsibility to advocate for yourself. If you don't, who will?

▸ *As the patient, you should feel comfortable with all members of your oncology team.* If there's someone with whom you don't feel at ease, speak up. Being comfortable helps your recovery.

▸ *Don't leave the office until you feel like you have a full understanding of everything that was discussed.*

Ask my doctor

What the patient needs to know: A sampling of questions to build upon

What's my prognosis? _____

_____

Where can I get more information on my diagnosis? _____

_____

_____

How do I go about getting a second opinion? _____

_____

_____

What stage am I in? What does that mean? _____

_____

What grade am I? What does that mean? _____

_____

What are my treatment options? Pros and cons of each? _____

_____

_____

_____

If you were in my place, what would you do? _____

_____

_____

Tell me about the side effects of the treatment(s). _____

_____

_____

What can I do to minimize the side effects? Nutrition? Medication?

Sleeping? Vitamins? _____

_____

_____

_____

Will this be covered by insurance? _____

What non-surgical options could I utilize? _____

_____

What about alternative medicines? _____

_____

What about nutritional alternatives? _____

_____

_____

How many lymph nodes really need to be removed? What kind of testing

can be done before? _____

_____

What physical restrictions will I be facing? _____

_____

_____

How long will I need to be off work? Will I have any restrictions? _____

_____

_____

What signs or symptoms of recurrence or other problems should I look for?

52

_____

_____

What kind of activities or exercises will speed my recovery? _____

_____

_____

What are my plastic surgery options? _____

_____

What information do you have at your office on support groups for

myself, my family? _____

_____

How often do I need to come in to see you? _____

_____

_____

_____

_____

_____

_____

_____

_____

_____

"Be confident & firm with your doctors. Ask lots of questions."
Diane, 47, breast

Checklist

Things I can or should do before I enter the hospital

Who needs to be notified?

- ☐ _____
- ☐ _____
- ☐ _____
- ☐ _____
- ☐ _____
- ☐ _____

What do I need to cancel or take care of immediately?

- ☐ _____
- ☐ _____
- ☐ _____
- ☐ _____

Who can help take care of children, spouse, parent, etc?

- ☐ _____
- ☐ _____
- ☐ _____
- ☐ _____
- ☐ _____
- ☐ _____

Busy work but important

- ☐ Make phone and address list to take with me
- ☐ Write cards ahead of time for children, significant other, etc.
- ☐ Are all the proper papers in order, i.e. living will, advance directives
- ☐ Discuss "do not resuscitate" code status
- ☐ Pre-plan any emergency
- ☐ Prepare phone list to keep close by at all times
- ☐ _____
- ☐ _____
- ☐ _____
- ☐ _____
- ☐ _____
- ☐ _____
- ☐ _____

Checklist

Things I need from home while I'm in the hospital

Clothing

- ☐ Underwear
- ☐ Socks
- ☐ Sweatpants
- ☐ Sweater
- ☐ Scarf
- ☐ _____
- ☐ _____
- ☐ _____

Personal items

- ☐ Toothbrush, toothpaste
- ☐ Hair brush
- ☐ Lotion
- ☐ Eyeglasses, contacts
- ☐ Make up
- ☐ Pillow
- ☐ Medications
- ☐ _____
- ☐ _____
- ☐ _____
- ☐ _____

Extras

Pictures
- ☐ _____
- ☐ _____

Music CDs, tapes
- ☐ _____
- ☐ _____
- ☐ _____

Books
- ☐ _____
- ☐ _____

Magazines
- ☐ _____
- ☐ _____

Newspapers
- ☐ _____
- ☐ Journal
- ☐ Pens and paper
- ☐ Phone numbers, addresses
- ☐ _____
- ☐ _____

Ask the doctor

What the caregiver needs to know: A sampling of questions to build upon

Ask these types of questions if permitted by patient. These can help clarify a lot of information.

What does the diagnosis mean? _____

_____

What's the prognosis and what does that mean? _____

_____

How can we find more information? _____

_____

_____

What do we need from you in getting a second opinion, i.e. x-rays, tests?

_____

_____

Is the treatment offered locally? If not, where? _____

_____

_____

How long will he/she be hospitalized? _____

_____

over

What are the side effects of the treatment(s)? _____

_____

When should we seek immediate medical attention? _____

_____

56

What training do I need to take care of dressings, drains, etc.?_____

_____

Will this affect her/his emotional well-being? How can I help? _____

_____

_____

What physical activities should he/she avoid? How long? _____

_____

_____

At what point should he/she resume more activity? _____

_____

How do we get necessary forms for medical leave? _____

_____

Who else can we talk to in the office if you're not here? _____

_____

Who do we contact on weekends and holidays? _____

_____

Who can we talk to about support groups? _____

_____

Where can we go for additional assistance? _____

_____

_____

Talking about treatment...

▶ If surgery is needed, get the best surgeon there is. *N, 80, breast*

▶ I'm sure they have been told the statistics by the doctors. I would prepare them for what to expect in terms of side effects. *Joseph, 25, Hodgkin's lymphoma*

▶ Look for alternative treatments. *Ralph, 68, prostate*

▶ Get a good doctor and read about the particular cancer you have. Get as much info as can be found. *Murray, 64, lymphoma*

▶ Something that I would have liked is to have had someone research the latest options and the latest statistics regarding the cancer and procedure that I had. *Julie, 61, breast*

▶ I couldn't believe at 92 someone could get breast cancer! *L, 65, best friend, breast*

▶ Just because there are treatment options available, it might not be right for your loved one. Pray about every decision. Look for the options that will give the best quality of life. Remember, quality is more important than quantity. *Lisa, 40, husband, brain*

▶ She was very outspoken with all doctors and involved in her treatment phases. *Liz, 43, sister, breast*

▶ I wanted to go to other institutions for other treatments. *Ralph, 68, wife, breast*

▶ Complete trust in my doctors and my faith. *Linda, 62, breast*

▶ We both believed being armed with information was more important. *Mary, 52, husband, kidney*

▶ My great oncologist along with the whole oncology/hematology floor. Entering through those double doors and seeing and feeling the love and comfort they have was such a great comfort to me. I felt I was never going to lose. *Nancy, 57, non-Hodgkins lymphoma*

▸ My cancer is not your friend's cousin's brother. All our diagnoses, treatments and responses are different. *Diane, 38, thyroid*

▸ He took notes and helped me absorb what the doctor said. I seemed to forget quickly what the doctor said. *D, 42, breast*

▸ Always assure individual they are in control of treatment. *P, 62, husband, throat and neck*

▸ Get second doctor's opinion. *Ralph, 68, prostate*

▸ Reading up and understanding where I was with my cancer. Discovering it with my doctors. *Mary, 64, breast*

▸ I kept a daily diary so I could tell the doctor how he was responding to the chemo and medicine. It helped a great deal. One dosage of medication was changed. *Marianne, 71, husband, large cell lymphoma*

▸ Being a nurse, I asked the doctor a lot of questions. I also gave my husband questions to ask, too. *Mary, 48, husband, thyroid*

▸ Research all of your options through the Internet, second opinions, books, etc., and ask a lot of questions. *Diane, 47, breast*

▸ Always get a second opinion on diagnosis and treatment. *P, 62, husband, throat and neck*

▸ Be your own advocate and "push" to get what you feel you need. Be assertive and progressive. It's your life, after all. *Cheryl, 48, rectal*

▸ He was positive and strong in the beginning. Honest about diagnosis and prognosis. I am a nurse, so he knew I knew a lot of medical things. *C, 63, father, esophageal and liver*

"It never dawned on me that I would not get well."
Judith, 70, breast

For the record

What you need to know about me

Type of cancer _____

Oncologist _____

Phone number _____

Surgeon _____

Phone number _____

Family physician _____

Phone number _____

Back-up physician to call _____

Phone number _____

Pharmacy _____

Phone number _____

Address _____

Medications _____

Allergies _____

Current treatment _____

Location of schedule for medications _____

Symptoms to be concerned about _____

Hospital in case of emergency _____

Location of important paperwork _____

Hey Doc!

▸ Dad always looked forward to his doctor's visits. He always wanted to be a doctor, and he liked learning about medical things. *Abbie, 51, father, leukemia*

▸ Family physician had not sent friend for proper diagnostics (mammogram) as he "felt" it was a fibroid cyst. Delay in diagnosis was detrimental to patient's outcome. *Pam, friend, breast and lung*

▸ (I wish I had had) more training as to what effects the chemo has on the body. How to eat properly. *Jeannie, 60, breast*

▸ Mixed. Love. Not certain what to expect. Doctor had to be pinned down, not communicative, no prognosis given or what to expect. *Virginia, 66, husband, colon; mother-in-law, colon*

▸ After my biopsy, I met with a nurse who told me about my cancer and the next steps. We met for an hour. It seemed longer. She gave me too much information. It was overwhelming. She was talking mastectomy, and I was trying to deal with being told I have cancer. *D, 42, breast*

▸ Worst experience, telephone call from radiologist, "you have cancer." Second worse, surgeon said, "We'll remove your breast." When asked if this was necessary, he said it's no big deal. "You certainly at your age shouldn't care." I was 45. *S, breast*

▸ I would like to have known what my chances of survival were. *Betty, 75, breast*

▸ I was told radiation wouldn't hurt much, but it did. I haven't spoken to any who have had it that didn't agree. *Rita, 58, breast*

▸ The time that is given to a patient in an office or hospital is like being herded through a gate. *Barbara, 61, breast*

▸ Doctor was wonderful with his honest but hopeful attitude. *Judy, 65, breast*

▸ Frustrated and saddened that diagnosis was not more aggressive. Friend trusted the advice of her family physician and felt she was okay. *Pam, friend, breast and lung*

▸ My surgeon and chemo doctor were both very positive and always answered any questions or fears I had. *Karen, 62, breast*

▸ Honesty by doctors, nurses and family and the idea we were working together to fight this and hopeful outlook. *Mary Ann, 56, colorectal*

▸ I wish all the medical people involved in my care would have been more informative. I think they are busy, and you don't get the time and information you need. If you want information about having radiation or not, who do you go to? They only refer you to radiation oncologists, and of course, they're only going to tell you to go through with it because that's their profession. What about people who have gone through radiation and might have been better off if they hadn't gone through it? Where can you get that kind of information? *Shari, 50, breast*

61

▸ What would I tell doctors treating cancer patients? To be more personable, treat them as human beings, not as a patient. When giving the person the news and the person cries, don't yell at them. That happened to me. Why? Because I asked him the same question. I didn't even realize he was yelling at me. The person I was with told me he yelled at me. I got rid of him. I've had trouble with doctors because everyone wants to take charge, which is fine, but I want the best of both worlds because it's my life. I should have the right to have two doctors. They should be able to share. It's my life. If I want six doctors, then I'll use six doctors. It's also part of letting doctors know who's really the boss, and that's the patient. *D, 60, ovarian*

▸ My doctors were all incredible, brilliant, caring people. They saved my life. They had wonderful staff that cared deeply about you. I took their advice and chose the most aggressive treatment available. I believe this is one of the main reasons I am here today. The positive attitude was a big contributor as well. *Diane, 47, breast*

"The desire to take medicine is perhaps the greatest feature which distinguishes man from animals." Sir William Osler

Just one of many

62

- "I had my best friend stay with me while I was in the hospital. She was able to attend to all of the little things like getting me drinks, helping me to the bathroom, washing my face with a warm cloth and other things not as easily available due to nursing shortages."

- "I had friends and family bring up a large poster of my children, home, friends and lots of laughter and fun times. We put it on the wall, and nurses and visitors enjoyed it almost as much as I did."

- "I got a cute pair of warm pajamas from a friend that made me feel and look better and helped me to feel more comfortable while in the hospital."

- "I had a friend who came to the hospital and actually washed my hair with dry soap. Because of all my chest incisions, I needed to keep this area dry and couldn't stand the dirty hair. She also brought in some comfortable clothes, make up and a mirror to help me look and feel better."

- "Friends took up a collection to buy me a new wig. What an uplifting thing."

▸ "I had a friend who brought some wonderful lotion and gave me a relaxing back rub. I know you can't remember all of the nice things people do for you after surgery because of the medications, but I often think of that and how wonderful it was."

▸ "One thing people need to remember is to keep the visit short, especially if the patient is sleepy or is getting a lot of phone calls. A short hello will mean just as much and maybe even more appreciated than a longer stay."

▸ "I thought any small gift that was comforting, such as a pillow, blanket or even a basket of snacks was great."

▸ "It's just a disease. Don't give it more power or act like it is somehow the absolute worst thing. That may frighten your friend more."

▸ "I wanted people to know they could ask me anything. I still wanted to be viewed as approachable. I really wanted people to treat me as the same person."

▸ "You really have to stay away from negative people, can't afford to waste your time."

Robin's friends

64

Coping strategies

"Being deeply loved by someone gives you strength; loving someone deeply gives you courage."
Lao-Tzu

Survivors reveal useful coping mechanisms

We asked our survivors to select five coping mechanisms from a list of common coping strategies utilized by those who are experiencing massive traumatic stress. These coping mechanisms are typical means for human survival and resiliency, and hold powerful elements to assist our loved ones with their battle against cancer.

Recently, I (Miller, 2001) completed a similar survey with women who were interned in Auschwitz concentration camp during the Holocaust. Utilizing a sample of women who gave their testimony to the United States Holocaust Museum in Washington D.C., the research indicated that *love and affiliation with others* was the most prominent coping strategy for survival in Auschwitz.

In comparison, our cancer survey results show a similar correlation, indicating the *importance of affiliation with others as a means of coping, resiliency and survival*. Looking through the survey results, you can easily see the importance of friendship, family connection, and love in the perceived resiliency of cancer survivors.

Additionally, concurring with current research related to *survival and faith,* you will notice the large portion of our cancer survivors view their *faith and prayer* as a powerful coping technique in their survival.

Our cancer survey resoundingly noted the importance of prayer and faith, which was rated by most of our cancer survivors as one of their most important coping strategies. Close behind were issues highlighting the importance of love and connection (friendship, significant other's love and assistance from others) as a coping mechanism used for their survival. The chart on the following page will give you an overview of the results of our cancer survey.

But clearly our survivors view many other things as important in their ability to survive and thrive. Here are some of the other coping mechanisms our survivors noted in our survey results.

66

Coping technique	Incidence of usage
Prayer and faith	117
Love of a significant other	94
Hope of living to be with family & friends	78
Personal determination	65
Living one day at a time	57
Assistance from others	56
Friendships	55
Knowledge	47
Humor	46
Daily tasks or routines	37
Visualization and meditation	16
Creating choices	14
Purpose or meaning	14
Talking about the future	14
Maintaining dignity	12
Staying numb	6
Living for a specific event	6
Denial or resisting the reality of diagnosis	5
Luck or chance	4
Anger or rage	3

- Being able to continue my job … my ability to work
- Being able to witness and enjoy nature
- Having a task to focus upon
- Acceptance of my disease, as well as the acceptance from my loved ones
- Having a supportive and knowledgeable physician
- Assistance from a 12-step support group
- Reading inspirational books
- Recreation
- Being able to travel
- Hearing success stories
- Knowing that I had the security of a home that was warm and loving
- The love of my pets

- Being able to maintain a healthy lifestyle
- The constant love that surrounded me
- My determination
- Living for my grandchildren
- Lots of hugs from loved ones and friends
- Feeling needed despite my cancer diagnosis
- Listening to music
- A cancer center
- No longer being caught in anxiety and worry — seeing this as a waste of time and energy
- Humor and laughter
- Visits from fellow cancer survivors
- The desire to be a parent
- Helping others

- Obtaining knowledge about the cancer, treatment, and survival rates
- Practicing holistic health
- Doing crossword puzzles
- Sharing my experience to help educate others
- Journaling
- Serving as a role model
- Maintaining an exercise program
- Having faith in myself
- Staying occupied with hobbies and crafts
- Enjoying and experiencing nature
- Sharing feelings with loved ones
- Enjoying every moment as a "gift"
- Taking "control" of the cancer

Top responses

- Prayer and faith
- Love of a significant other
- Hope to live to be with family & friends
- Personal determination
- Living one day at a time
- Assistance from others
- Staying positive

A deeper look at coping

The understanding of the "nature of coping" is an essential part of human adaptation during the diagnosis of cancer or other life-threatening disorders. Facing the unknown, we fight for survival by attempting to find meaning, a purpose, and the will to take another breath to live.

Coping strategies have been the topic of volumes of research in the past 60 years. Our powerful ability to utilize coping strategies has been studied in World War II veterans, Vietnam veterans, Holocaust survivors, cancer survivors and other survivors of life-threatening trauma, as well as abuse victims.

Psychologist R.S. Lazarus (1991) believes coping consists of cognitive (psychological techniques) and behavioral (tasks) techniques, which help manage levels of stress. The two coping strategies are *problem-focused* (creating choices, doing daily tasks, etc.) and *emotion-focused* coping (hope, prayer, love, determination, etc.). Simply put, problem-focused coping is action-centered or "doing something," while emotion-focused coping involves thinking rather than acting/doing strategies.

Lazarus suggests that problem-focused and emotion-focused coping are utilized at differing degrees of stress. He proposes that at low degrees of stress, we use the two forms at an identical or similar frequency. At moderate range of perceived stress, problem-focused (doing a task) coping appears to be more prevalent. While at high levels of stress, such as cancer, emotion-focused coping appears to be the predominant coping strategy.

Consequently, in situations such as the cancer, there are few opportunities to utilize problem-focused coping strategies, limiting the utilization of that technique for adaptation. The survivor can look for various treatment options, but their ability to change the diagnosis is impossible.

Many times, survivors' problem-solving mechanisms depend on the competencies of their surgeons, treatment teams, and available medical options. The options are limited. Therefore, many cancer survivors have learned the importance of emotion-focusing coping mechanisms as a means of enhancing survival. These coping techniques involve psychological techniques such as one's faith, affiliation with friends or family, hope, and trying to find a meaning or purpose to continue living.

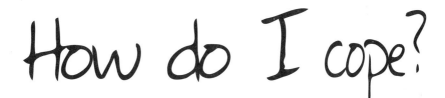
How do I cope?

For the patient/survivor: These pages will help you examine how you are coping with cancer. Pick your top 5

Assistance from others   _____

Hope of living to be with family & friends   _____

Prayer and faith   _____

Purpose or meaning   _____

Humor   _____

Staying numb   _____

Denial or resisting the reality of diagnosis   _____

Anger or rage   _____

Personal determination   _____

Talking about the future   _____

Love of a significant other   _____

Visualization and meditation   _____

Daily tasks or routines   _____

Creating choices   _____

Knowledge   _____

Living one day at a time   _____

Luck or chance   _____

Friendships   _____

Maintaining dignity   _____

Living for a specific event   _____

over

How do I cope overall? _____

_____

_____

_____

What techniques seem to work best for me and why? _____

_____

_____

_____

_____

Which coping strategies can be harmful for me (i.e., denial, not facing reality, overworking to ignore reality, etc.) and why? _____

_____

_____

_____

_____

What problem-focused techniques can I use and how? _____

_____

_____

_____

What emotion-focused techniques can I use and how? _____

_____

_____

_____

_____

_____

"Simply accepting it. Lots of people get cancer."
Betty, 68, breast

Survivors say...

Were there other things that helped you cope and thrive?

Physical

▸ I worked every day up to my surgery date. At least I was busy, not that you ever stop thinking about it. *Robin, 46, breast*

▸ I told everyone about the diagnosis and what I wanted from them, funny cards, not preachy, and to ask anything they wanted to know. *Karen, 62, breast*

▸ Lots of sleep and music. *Maria, 61, breast*

▸ Bringing me books to read, buying me a wig after I lost all my hair. *Alveretta, 85, ovarian*

▸ Trying to maintain my same routine, work, etc. *Bill, 64, throat and tongue*

▸ I tried to maintain a healthy lifestyle, continue as normal as possible and keep a positive attitude. *Judith, 70, breast*

▸ We remodeled our kitchen, planned it, did it, lived through the mess. It helped to avoid thinking about illness! *Jeannie, 60, breast*

▸ When I was first diagnosed, I was working at a nursing home as a CNA. I felt very needed as a caregiver in my job, so I had no time for self pity. *Vicki, 53, breast*

▸ My husband was in fourth stage of colon cancer, and I needed to take care of him. *Linda, 62, breast*

▸ Desire to pass my estate in better order. *Joseph, 80, bladder*

▸ My animals and the support of a certain doctor. *Yvonne, 74, breast*

▸ I was asked to help at my old job for a few days, even though I had to wear a hat. Great morale booster. *Dorothy, 70, breast*

▸ A stranger gave me a bear to hug. *C, 79, breast*

▸ Rest at home. Sitting in my yard. *Dona, 74, NA*

Emotional

▸ Healing masses. *Mary, 62, breast*

▸ Wanting to see grandchildren grow. *John, 81, prostate and colon*

▸ I had just lost my mother three weeks before being diagnosed. She had suffered numerous strokes over nearly a year. When she was dying, I told her it was okay to let go. After that, how could I be afraid of anything. *Rita, 58, breast*

▸ People calling and keeping in touch, and prayers. Knowing I was in prayers or on prayer lists at different churches. *Mary Ann, 56, colon*

▸ The compassion and kindness I found at the Cancer Center, a soft place to fall! Thank you! *Paula, 53, uterine and breast*

▸ Positive attitude. Being "too mean" to let it get me. *Judy, 56, breast*

▸ Hearing success stories from other survivors. *Theresa, 49, breast*

▸ Good doctors. *G, 57, endometrial*

▸ The care and compassion of friends. *Diane, 47, breast*

▸ Having cancer survivors call me and tell me of their experiences. *Martha, 51, breast*

▸ All the "life" that surrounds me, realizing that I neglected it before and now realizing I'm not ready to give it up. *Sara, 35, lung*

▸ Just the determination that I wasn't going to let cancer win. I have too much to live for, and I knew that having a positive attitude was part of the battle. *Melinda, 46, breast*

▸ Plan to have a good day! *JoAnn, breast*

▸ A visit from Robin Unes, just the look of understanding, empathy and compassion in her eyes. *Diane, 38, thyroid*

"Where there is love there is life." Mahatma Gandhi

72

How family and friends view survivors' coping

We decided to ask our significant others, friends, and family to evaluate what they viewed as the coping mechanism used by their loved one who was diagnosed with cancer. You will quickly see that our caregivers/family/friends actually had almost *identical* results to the survivors' responses. Placed in a different order, but assessing the same coping techniques as important to survival and thriving, both the survivors and our caregivers/family/friends chose: *faith/prayer, personal determination, love of a significant other, and hope of being with family and friends, and living one day at a time,* as essential to their resiliency and thriving.

Coping technique	Incidence of usage
Faith or prayer	97
Personal determination	81
Love of significant others	77
Hope of living to be with family, friends,	71
Taking one day at a time	54
Humor	43
Daily tasks/routine	43
Knowledge	43
Assistance from others	42
Friendships	40
Maintaining dignity	35
Talking about the future	30
Purpose or meaning	21
Denial or resisting reality of the diagnosis	14
Visualization/meditation	13
Living for a specific event	13
Staying numb	9
Anger or rage	9
Creating choices	8
Luck	4

How others watched the patient/survivor cope

74

- Caring for a pet
- Staying active by volunteering
- Having wonderful hospice nurses
- Having the love of family
- Maintaining a positive attitude
- Making amends with family or friends
- Prayer and faith
- The desire to live or to live their last days to their fullest
- Maintaining a "normal" life
- Staying involved with the arts (music, books, writing)
- Living to be with grand-children
- The constant presence of family and friends
- Knowledge you have lived a full life
- Feeling some control because you can plan your own funeral
- The ability to be able to pass possessions down to loved ones as a means of saying goodbye

- Laughter and humor
- The ability to question and interact with doctors
- Maintaining a healthy living program (alternative diet, exercise, vitamins, massages)
- Raising children
- Denial
- Taking care of someone else (aging parent or grandchild)
- Attending support groups
- Talking about feelings
- Interaction with others that have same diagnosis
- The family's acceptance of the disease
- E-mailing
- Helping others in similar situations cope with their illness
- Shaving their head and beating cancer to the punch
- Knowledge we've taken the most aggressive treat-ment possible

Loved ones say...

What other things helped the patient/survivor cope or thrive?

Physical

▸ She took great pride in her work. Her personal relationships at work were important. Her job was also her only source of income, very important! *Sharon, 65, friend, breast*

▸ Gardening. When she could no longer garden outside, she transplanted hostas inside in her kitchen the fall before she died in January. *Nancy, 67, mother, pancreatic*

▸ Exercise, being asked by others for help. My son asked for my father's help finding a used car. It took his mind off things and made him feel useful, which he is! *Laura, 44, father, prostate*

▸ Raising children. *Jean, 64, mother, cervical*

▸ Reading, writing, music. *Phyllis, 59, friend, prostate*

▸ Volunteer work at her church. *Laura, 44, aunt, lymph*

▸ Spending time watching or playing with our babies (four years and one year old when he died), watching TV, Cubs games. *Monica, 35, husband, pancreatic*

▸ Mom enjoyed going to lunch with her close friends. They would show up and take her on a date about once a week. Mom's dog was her joy, too. *Rue, 29, mother, breast*

▸ Listening to CDs of sounds of nature, etc. Seemed to help with sleep. *Patti, 52, husband, RCC*

Emotional

▸ To know that I (his wife) survived cancer. *Patricia, 64, husband, larynx*

▸ His wonderful attitude in life in general. After coping with cancer three times, he was determined to lick it yet again. *Marianne, 71, husband, large cell lymphoma*

▸ Never complaining. *Lois, 53, mother, breast*

- Yes, the fact that I accepted it. *Ron, 62, wife, breast*
- He has Down Syndrome so it was hard to tell. *Judi, 64, son, leukemia*
- Unfortunately, my sister resisted going to the doctor and the denial of anything wrong resulted in her being very sick when she knew there was something wrong 10-12 months earlier. *Rosemary, 66, sister, ovarian*
- Lots of help from professionals, support from family. *Barbara, 66, husband, larynx*
- Mostly accepted the fact that she made the decision to smoke although she knew the consequences. Father died the same way. *Len, 51, sister, lung*
- Help from family, friends and hospice nurses. Being able to be at home clear until the end. *Tracy, 47, mother, lung*
- Assisting and aiding others through their cancer journey. *Leonard, 41, wife, breast*
- A plan to get life in order for those left behind, including planning her own funeral. *Pam, friend, breast and lung*
- Her positive attitude contributed largely. Also, things like shaving her head instead of watching it fall out. Helping others dealing with the same situation. *Kathleen, 24, mother, breast*
- She would use every bit of energy to make her children optimistic. *Tilley, 72, daughter, breast*
- She tried to identify and let go of stressors that were not good for her health and well-being. *Lori, 39, partner, breast*

" Challenges are what make life interesting; overcoming them is what makes life meaningful."
Joshua J. Marine

Caregivers sometimes need to apply a little tough love

Patti had to occasionally adopt some tough love tactics to keep her husband focused during his treatment for cancer of the kidney and brain.

She recalls how he called her a couple of times at work and announced he wasn't going in for treatment that day. She knew he had been overwhelmed by the battle, but she displayed enough courage to speak up and get him back on track again. Laughing, she admits she probably "came across as a bitch" at times, but she knew when to tell him what to do, and he'd do it.

Her husband had to give up the control of his life to cancer, and that was an intense challenge for both of them. She remembers how they both cried in Texas, where he was being treated. He wanted to come home, period, but she fought to keep him focused on his care.

At the same time, she describes the man she married as "unbelievably wonderful" as he has tackled both the physical and emotional toll of cancer. She's been with him during the painful moments and hours and encouraged him as he researched more about his disease and treatment options. However, he's also had to learn how his cancer has affected the entire family, how his frustration has turned into being short-tempered at times with their children.

"It's not been easy," she adds.

Patti explains that it's also been difficult for them because some people look at him and don't "see" anything wrong, so they find it hard to believe he's sick as he experienced a recurrence of cancer, this time in the brain. Family and friends have offered support at a level they would have never imagined.

He goes to a support group, which helps. Patti laughingly notes how a female cancer patient needed a ride to meetings, so he offered to help her, yet made it clear that he was a married man and wasn't hitting on her.

Sometimes he apologizes to Patti for what has happened to him and the extra demands placed upon her. However, she always reminds him with a loving, "Have you heard me complaining?"

Lesson #1
Sometimes you have to motivate the survivor

Assisting loved ones with coping

Cancer effects everyone who loves the survivor. In an effort to assist their family and friends, our survivors compiled a list of tips to assist their loved ones.

▶ Keep a sense of humor
▶ Remember to address your feelings of grief
▶ Join a cancer support group
▶ Give unconditional love to your survivor and to each other
▶ Show your feelings and emotions
▶ Maintain a positive affirming attitude
▶ Think in terms of recovery
▶ Maintain self care through good nutrition
▶ Be self loving and get plenty of sleep and exercise to help deal with the stressful situation
▶ Be open and honest
▶ Don't dwell on the cancer
▶ Tell your loved one how much you love them
▶ Show acceptance
▶ Be empathetic and compassionate
▶ Pray
▶ Remind yourself of the positives and small steps of accomplishment
▶ Be involved
▶ Communicate!
▶ Remind yourself about your inner strength and affirm your power to handle this adversity
▶ Help with routine tasks
▶ Remember that people love you and are there for you to lean on

"My teenage son thinks Grandpa walks on water. Grandpas and grandkids can be great therapy for everyone!"
Laura, 44, father, prostate

- Reach out to others for assistance
- Try to maintain somewhat of a normal aspect in your life
- Be patient with your survivor and yourself
- Try not to smother your survivor because they need to feel responsible and capable
- Let friends help
- Allow yourself the gift of crying
- Give lots of hugs
- Listen to positive people and stay away from negative influences
- Stay busy
- Obtain assistance from cancer centers or support groups
- Accept that all your emotions are normal
- Be understanding

- Remember the importance of knowledge
- Acknowledge that many people don't know how to assist, so be specific in suggesting how they might help
- Remember it is not your job to protect people from the truth, so be honest about the reality of the situation and your needs
- Realize this is a confusing time for you and be gentle with yourself
- Take time to spend some extra time with your children
- Make sure you take time to get away from the hospital
- Remember you have to care for yourself so you can be there for your loved one

Top responses

- Stay positive and affirming
- Keep a sense of humor
- Show acceptance
- Pray
- Listen listen listen

Everybody's body responds differently to cancer

"Yes, I had to have chemo and radiation, and the lymph nodes were taken, so I eventually developed a mild case of lymphedema. But I was never sick with the chemo, never sick from the radiation, healed quickly from surgery, and I felt like a fraud when I know people are looking at me admiringly for being 'so strong,' how they then say something about how proud they are of me for going through everything so well. I never thought, 'Why me?' I take it for granted that God would never send illness or a disease as a punishment. When I was first diagnosed, that night I asked God for strength to get through whatever was ahead, and I had it immediately. I would be devastated if I ever have to go through it all again, I know that. But, at the same time, I feel as I have had it so easy compared to so many others." Karen, 62, breast

Listen to me!

"All people want is someone to listen."
Hugh Elliott

Reaching loved ones: Keys to effective communication

We're quite confident that you would like to communicate effectively with your loved one, but perhaps you don't feel like you have the skills. Well, the most important element of effective communication is your desire to really "hear" what the other person is trying to say. Your desire to "know" what is inside their mind, their heart, and their soul is easily recognized by your loved one — and that's half the challenge.

In an attempt to enhance your skill level you will find some tips below. These are proven techniques that will enhance any relational conversation, especially with those you love!

Keys to effective communication with your loved one include:

▸ *Dedicate yourself to the conversation.* This means you are totally aware of the importance of the communication, and the energy that is required in the exchange. This may sound silly, but how many times have you caught yourself half listening to someone during a conversation? Effectively listening to your loved one means you are giving them your full attention.

▸ *Use "active listening techniques."* These techniques include effective body language (leaning forward, smiling, uncrossing your arms, nodding), which conveys that you really want to open the line of communication with your loved one.

▸ *A majority of communication is silent.* Researchers estimate that approximately one half of our communication is expressed through body language or facial expressions. Effectively communicating with your loved one means you are cognizant of body gestures, posture and breathing, which indicate meaning. For instance, your loved one may say they don't want to talk, but their eyes or non-verbal messages may indicate quite the opposite.

▸ *Paraphrase what you hear.* Make sure you understand what your loved one is conveying by paraphrasing what they have said to you. This tells your loved one that you really understand what they have said, and that you are actively interested in their thoughts and feelings.

▶ *Remember to listen with your heart as well as your ears.* Really listening to your loved one means that you open your heart and hear their thoughts, feelings, and the depth of their conversation. Listening with your heart also means you are willing to open yourself to your own feelings, and are willing to convey those feelings to your loved one.

▶ *Be emphatic.* Try to listen and ask yourself, "How can I hear my loved one's feelings and show I understand?" Empathy is communicated to your loved one through simple gestures as nods, or saying things such as, " I understand," "I know you are fearful," "I can really hear you are unsure about treatment options."

▶ *Make sure you are really "open" to the conversation.* Effective listening necessitates your own willingness to be open to conversation. If you aren't ready to devote yourself to the conversation, wait and find a time when you can be 100 percent dedicated to your loved one.

▶ *Try to be positive.* Effective communication involves trying to understand your loved one through loving eyes. Remember how devastating it can be if your loved one believes you are critical of their decisions, life choices, thoughts and feelings.

▶ *Use encouragement.* Many cancer patients report they need to hear their loved ones talk about their personal power to beat cancer, live with dignity, or how they are a model of strength to so many others.

▶ *Stay on target.* Remember to stay focused on the conversation. Your loved one needs to know you are willing to listen and not wander onto unrelated topics.

▶ *Keep an open mind.* Be conscious of not pushing your loved one away by dismissing their feelings, critiquing their decisions, or telling them how they should think or feel.

▶ *Be aware of pseudo-listening.* Be cautious of the message you send to your loved one if you look interested, but are concentrating on another subject, looking off into space, or hearing only part of what is being communicated. Be aware that pseudo-listening gives the message you are rejecting your loved one.

▶ *Maintain effective eye contact.* Nothing is worse than opening your heart to someone and noticing they are watching a television show while you are trying to discuss something important. Let your loved one know you are "with them" by maintaining eye contact and nodding occasionally when they speak.

▶ *Remember effective communication can be aided by an occasional touch.* A simple touch of the hand, or a hug can let your loved one know you are hearing everything they are saying and accepting and love them. Remember that your loved one might be struggling with feelings that their body has turned against them, or feel embarrassed about transformations that have occurred during treatment (loss of hair, losing a breast, impotency, weight gain). A simple touch can be a transformational gesture of love.

▶ *Your physical closeness to your loved one illustrates you want to communicate.* Anthropologist Edward Hall believes the closer you are in proximity to your loved one, the more intimate the conversation and relationship. Putting physical distance between you and your loved one indicates nonverbally that you want barriers in your relationship.

▶ *Really listen versus preparing your next statement.* An effective listener is focused on their loved one, instead of mentally preparing their own thoughts and rebuttal to the loved one's words.

▶ *If your loved one seems anxious and fearful, try techniques to help them be calm.* One method to aid communication with someone who is fearful is to slow down the speed of your conversation. Add a gentle touch, slow down your breathing, or speak in a quieter voice, and you will notice their anxiety and fear is lessened.

▶ *Be affirming.* Use nods to show you are listening. Say things like "uh huh," or "tell me more about that," or "I really want to understand a little better — please explain."

▶ *Notice gentle cues.* If your loved one starts to look downward, realize they are telling you something that comes from their heart. Be attentive and don't miss the importance of their conversation. Whatever they are saying at this time is very dear to their heart.

▶ *Think about what really matters.* Time is valuable, and cancer is not predictable. Remember there is nothing more pressing than "this moment" with your loved one.

Listening skills

- Stay focused on them
- Watch body language
- Keep eye contact; be close
- Listen with your heart!

How can I be a better communicator?

- _____
- _____
- _____
- _____
- _____
- _____

Active listening: Good listeners are not born, they master the skills

It's imperative to repeat that *listening is not a passive activity.* Effective listening takes energy, perseverance, attention, and consciously being "actively" engaged in the process.

Perhaps you are sitting here thinking, "Anyone can be a good listener. What's so hard about that?" Trust us, active listening is much more difficult than most people believe. Don't believe us? Take a moment and reflect. Think of a recent occasion in your life when you were trying to explain an important concept, or express a deep feeling to someone, and the listener just didn't understand you. There is nothing more hurtful and disturbing than feeling like someone doesn't actually "hear" what you have to say, or understand the true essence of what moves you.

It is essential that you understand how important listening is to the survivor. Filled with a plethora of thoughts and emotions, our loved ones want us to fully capture their true feelings and thoughts.

Active listening is somewhat like a metaphor of an iceberg. So, what does an iceberg have to do with your loved one? When you see a mammoth iceberg in the ocean you believe you are seeing the entire structure, but realistically you are only viewing 5 percent of the entity — 95 percent of the iceberg is hidden from your view. This is the perfect analogy! When you talk to your loved one, you are probably only hearing a small part of what they are trying to express to you.

So many of us forget that communication is not only verbal in nature, to the greatest degree, much of the discussion that is never uttered out loud is spoken non-verbally. So you can easily see that under the surface, your loved one is attempting to express so many feelings and emotions, but their words are only part of the communication. There's 95 percent of communication that just isn't expressed with words. Without understanding how to be an active listener, it's certain you will miss a great portion of their meaning without your knowledge.

Here are some key concepts to help you in your journey to lovingly listen actively with your survivor:

▶ *Watch for non-verbal communication.* Be aware of eye movement and facial cues. Here's an example: If you watch someone talk about the past their eyes tend to move to the left ... they are looking into reflections of what was. When you see someone's eyes look to the right and upward, they are looking to the future and hopeful! When someone looks down, they are dealing with their feelings, and when they look straight up, they generally are "in their head" and dealing with cognitive thoughts.

▶ *Watch for non-verbal body cues.* Are their arms crossed? This might mean they are defensive or keeping distant from you. Perhaps their legs are crossed away from you? This may also mean they are keeping you at a distance and not engaging with you. It's important to be aware of not only your loved one's non-verbal, but also your own. You may believe you want to listen to your survivor, but if you are turned sideways and away from the speaker, with your eyes darting around the room, while writing a list of things to do ... trust me, your loved one will most definitely never share an intimate feeling with you!

▶ *Try to "hear" the emotion, mood, fears or concerns in their unspoken word.* Your loved one might not tell you what they are really feeling, but you will be able to "read" those feelings if you are a skilled listener. You have to look beyond the words. Listen to the inflection of their voice. Try to hear the tone of their feelings. You have to trust your hunches. You have to clear your mind of clutter and try to "be with them" and visualize how they are feeling. In some ways it's like trying to get inside their skin and be part of every breath. This takes practice, but once you get skilled at this technique you will be able to "feel it" when it occurs. Let us caution you, that it is imperative to check out your hunches or perceptions, and not rely on being a mind reader. The way you will know if you are skilled at this technique is when you can reflect back a feeling or concept to your survivor and they tell you that you fully understand their message. Here are some examples of ways to phrase your reflection:
  • *"Are you really feeling scared, but having a hard time expressing it?"*
  • *"You say things are okay, but I look at your face and it appears you are anxious."*
  • *"Are you saying what you really want?"*

▶ *Listen in an attempt to validate.* A good listener is focused on the messages of the speaker, with the goal of respecting and validating their thoughts and feelings. Our survivors need to believe they are competent and capable of making good decisions and need someone to believe in them. Don't fall into the most common pitfall and look for what's wrong in your loved one's statements or feelings. Stay away from weaknesses, negative responses, and faults, and focus on the "real meaning" of what they are trying to say. Focus on respecting their point of view, and they will know that you really understand them.

▶ *Don't forget that men and women do talk in different languages.* Don't believe it? Well, just ask a man, "Could you take out the garbage?" To a man, you are asking, "Is it possible for you to take out the garbage?" Of course, he thinks, "I have the ability to take out the garbage!" But, to a woman, that sentence means, "Could you please take out the garbage ... *now!*" Of course, that isn't what she said, but her request is intrinsically a female understanding of, "If I said it, I would like some immediacy in the action." Remember men are typically problem solvers in their conversational style, and women talk as a means of sorting out their own solutions. So make sure you are talking the same language with your loved one. Ask questions to clarify meanings of words, thoughts, and impressions. It's better to check things out for clarity than mistakenly fall into miscommunication.

▶ *Focus on listening to your loved one, instead of your response.* Track the conversation and try to stay out of the clutter of your own mind and your response to immediately jump in and discuss things from your own viewpoint. An active listener keeps pace with the speaker by listening, reflecting back feelings, making clarifications and using non-verbal responses (like nodding, saying "ah-ha" and touching). Think of a tennis game. The key to active listening is to stay in your own court, and try not to dominate the game. If you really want to have a good long volley, you want to "hit" the ball to your loved one so they can feel like they are a valuable part of the game. Then you both can enjoy the pleasures of each other.

▶ *Learn to paraphrase.* When your loved one speaks to you, try to restate what they just said to you in different words. Typically, a therapist uses sentences like,"What I hear you saying is ..." or "If I understand you ..." This may seem like a silly little game,

▸ Don't ask, "Did they get it all?"

▸ Do not talk about all the side effects unless the survivor opens the conversation and wants to discuss them openly

▸ Do not call others and tell them about the diagnosis without the permission of the survivor

▸ Do not detach from the survivor — help them with the burden by showing support and love

▸ Do not make jokes about the impending loss (of body parts)

▸ Do not say, "Well, you probably won't be here much longer"

▸ Respect the survivor if they are not in the mood to talk

▸ Do not say, "I did this, or that…" Just listen

▸ Do not pretend it isn't happening

▸ Do not say, "How long did the doctor give you to live?"

▸ Do not ask, "Are you sure the doctor knows what he's doing?"

▸ Do not say, "Well, it's probably a misdiagnosis"

▸ Do not say, "Is this serious? Are you going to die?"

▸ Do not minimize the diagnosis

▸ Do not tell the survivor how to feel, think or how to act

▸ Do not say negative things about the survivor's choice of physicians — just be supportive and encouraging

> *When you are with a survivor, don't complain about your job, your life, or how bad things are going for you.*

▸ Do not say, "There must be a reason this is happening"

▸ Do not attack treatment choices made by your loved one.

▸ Do not attack your loved one's coping mechanisms (using humor, faith, denial, etc.)

▸ Do not offer false hope

▸ Do not make generalized offers such as: "Call if you need me." Trust us, they won't call. Remember that many loved ones don't want to be a burden, or don't know how to ask for assistance.

▸ Do not just talk about the cancer and nothing else

91

- Do not take it personally if you hear the loved one talk about anger, hurt, disappointment, etc. Remember, their feelings are not directed towards you.
- Do not deny the reality of the cancer
- Do not compare your loved one's illness to a cat or a dog who has cancer or a life-threatening illness

92

- Do not quote negative statistics or survival times
- Do not try to convert your loved one's religious beliefs and shove your own religious concepts on them. Listen and be supportive while nurturing your loved one's spiritual faith.
- Do not stare at the missing breast and not your loved one's face while talking
- Do not make comment about increases in weight, body puffiness, or wigs

Top responses

- Don't tell horror stories about other cancer patients
- Don't say, I know how you feel
- Don't pity them for their diagnosis
- Don't act like they're dying
- Don't say, it will be okay

My response

Survivor, family or friend:
How do I communicate?

What is the easiest way for me to communicate with my loved ones

and friends? Talk? Write? Physically? Other? Why?

_____

_____

_____

Am I or have I been afraid to express my emotions? Why?

_____

_____

_____

What do I want to say? _____

_____

_____

What do I want to ask? _____

_____

How can I keep the dialogue going? _____

_____

_____

_____

Survivors say...

What would you suggest someone NOT say or do when someone they know is diagnosed with cancer?

▶ Do not be a know-it-all about cancer. Each person is different and unique. *Tracy, 33, cervical*

▶ I hated it when someone said I was looking well, when I was losing weight, losing my hair, vomiting, not able to eat because of chemo. *Judith, 70, breast*

▶ "Oh you poor thing." Don't whine, don't act like I'm dying. *S, 61, breast*

▶ "Okay, they can cure that nowadays. It will be no problem." *Elaine, 72, leukemia*

▶ "How long did the doctor give you? Are you sure the doctor knows what he's doing?" *Donna, 72, colon*

▶ Do not start talking about other people who had cancer, treatments, or died ... yikes! *Maria, 61, breast*

▶ They should not want every medical detail, telling the "story" to everyone is depressing. *Jim, 50, thyroid*

▶ Keep thoughts positive, not discourage them in word or deed. *John, 81, prostate and colon*

▶ "I know how you feel." No, they don't. *N, 80, breast*

▶ Don't take offense at their moods. *Karen, 33, breast*

▶ "It is going to be okay." No one knows that. "Things will be fine." *Judy, 56, breast*

▶ Put blame on anyone for their condition. *Marilyn, 72, breast*

▶ Be calm. Do not alarm with too much information. *Marlene, 72, breast*

▶ "It's no big deal" or "You'll be fine." *Joseph, 25, Hodgkin's lymphoma*

▶ Don't pity the person. *Julie, 61, breast*

- Don't start crying. Don't act like you don't care. Don't try to stay away from the person. *Martha, 51, breast*

- Don't say, "Thank God it isn't me. I had a lump just like that. Thank God it wasn't cancer." *Helen, 72, lung*

- Don't avoid the person just because they have a disease. *Sara, 35, lung*

- I had a family member call one of my childhood friends and tell her. That really upset me. I felt that was my place to do that in my own time. *Noreen, 49, breast*

95

- Do not avoid your friend, cry with them! Share your heart. *Jeannie, 60, breast*

- "Oh, it's a breeze, nothing to it." *Carol, 71, colon*

- Don't give me a dead stare like I'm doing something wrong to have the pain I do without direction. This had happened to me in a doctor's office. *Barbara, 61, breast*

- Never be negative! There is always hope. When my cancer came back five years later, someone said to me, "I heard that you'll probably have recurrence every five years." Very stupid to say. *Vicki, 53, breast*

- Don't be blatantly pessimistic or blithely optimistic. *Clair, 55, breast*

> "I remember being in a department store, obviously bald, and the saleswoman couldn't even look at me." Ann, 45, breast

- I was only angry once, before surgery, right after diagnosis. I received an e-mail from someone who was a cancer survivor, a friend of a friend, who I didn't know. She did everything wrong: Told me she knew exactly how I felt and went on to say how much she cried and asked "Why me?" none of which I had done. She told me about how she'd lost her hair for nine months and now she was getting perms and color treatments, and then told me that if I would send her my address, she would send me the journal she wrote about her experiences. I didn't even know if I was going to have chemo, yet, I was so furious with this person. She was completely self-centered, breezy and obnoxious. *Karen, 62, breast*

Just one of many

Have any of these thoughts crossed your mind....

▸ Okay, now what should I do? My close friend has just been diagnosed with cancer.

▸ I kind of want to call, but what if she doesn't want to talk?

▸ Maybe I should stop over, but he may be resting.

▸ Maybe I'll call some more friends, find out what they know and do what they do.

▸ Maybe I won't call anyone and hope this is a mistake and it all blows over.

▸ Maybe if I don't say that "c" word, it couldn't possibly be true.

▸ Maybe he went to a quack doctor who is way off base. This is probably just a mix up.

▸ Well, surgery shouldn't be so bad. They go in, take it out, and this will be over.

▸ I didn't know this would mean surgery. How will she take off time from work, watch her kids?

▸ I call her husband, but he never wants any help.

▸ I just can't cope with surgery, that means blood and bandages. I wouldn't know how to act. I think I'll just wait until he's back at work and say something then.

97

- I wonder how sick she will be. I heard people look worse from the treatment than the cancer. Maybe I should wait to call until this is all over.

- I can't believe he has to do all this treatment now. They said the surgery would probably get it all. I wonder where his doctor went to school.

- How do I act when I see him next? Is he tired of hearing "how are you?" in the special, whispered voice?

- Does she still need any help with the kids or is all her energy back? Maybe help with the groceries or cleaning. Would it be an insult to offer?

- I imagine she wants to talk about this, and I want her to know I am here. Maybe I will drop by with some cookies and see if it is a good time.

- Now that the cancer is back, I wonder how long she has. I can't think of anything to say, I am so upset. I won't be able to even talk to her.

- All I can do is try to listen and be the strong one. I have to put her first and deal with my own stress at home.

- Everyone is calling me. Being the closest friend it seems like my phone never stops ringing. They all want to know what to do. How should I know?

- I just cannot cope with this. There is nothing I can do to make this better and I should probably distance myself at this point. She doesn't need help from someone who is scared to death.

Robin & friends

I wish someone...

We've given you some suggestions regarding what not to say or do, and hopefully, this will be a road map to help you through some difficult discussions with your loved one.

In a similar vein, our survivors made some remarkably simple suggestions about what they really wish someone had said to them, as well as some ideas for assistance they would have appreciated. Hopefully, this will give you a valuable insight into the secret thoughts of survivors.

▶ I wish someone would have helped me clean my house
▶ I wish someone would have weeded my garden
▶ I wish people would have brought over food
▶ I wish people would have been more light-hearted and humorous
▶ I wish someone would have said "this isn't the end of the world"
▶ I wish someone told me to "Get a second opinion"
▶ I wish my minister would have stopped by
▶ I wish people would have been more supportive of my fears
▶ I wish I knew about my chances for survival
▶ I wish my husband would have not been so sad and scared
▶ I wish someone would have discussed the options
▶ Instead of saying "let me know if I can help," say "I will do something specific" to help
▶ I wish someone had told me about the local cancer center
▶ I wish my daughter would have talked to me and given me hugs
▶ I wish some of my friends and family could cope better ... sat with me and just listened
▶ I wish my husband would have helped me and said everything would be all right
▶ I wish someone would have helped with my children
▶ I wish my husband was more understanding. He wanted things back to normal, which meant I was handling everything again
▶ I wish someone would have told me that treatment hurts
▶ I wish someone would have said, "You are cured"
▶ I wish my family was more informed

- I wish someone would let me talk about my cancer
- I wish I had the support of my work place
- I wish my siblings were supportive and loving to me
- I wish I was not kicked out of cancer treatment because the trials were finished ... this hurts more than anyone could know
- I wish my friends understood
- I wish someone would have told me what to expect after the mastectomy
- I wish someone had told me more about my specific condition
- I wish someone would have asked if I was afraid
- I wish someone had said, "Let it go, I'll be here to comfort you"
- I wish someone would have made me laugh
- I wish my physician was more holistic and emphasized a healthy diet
- I wish someone would have told me my hair would come back differently
- No one said "When chemotherapy is over, the pain may not be"
- I wish I knew what to expect from my doctor
- I wish the nurse or doctor would have called to check on me after my first chemotherapy
- I wish I had known a survivor with a similar condition
- I wish someone had talked about all the treatment options and the consequences of each
- I wish someone would have listened to my fears, my concerns, and offered some sympathy
- I wish I would have been prepared for the feelings I have — I have no support system
- I wish there was a support group for spouses
- I wish someone at work had shown some empathy
- I wish my friends had included me in activities, because I felt so shut out
- I wish someone close to me would have talked to me openly about my fear of dying

99

I wish some important people hadn't pretended there was no problem.

▶ I wish someone would have told me to focus on what I can do, vs. what I can't do

▶ I wish I had heard, "I love you!"

100

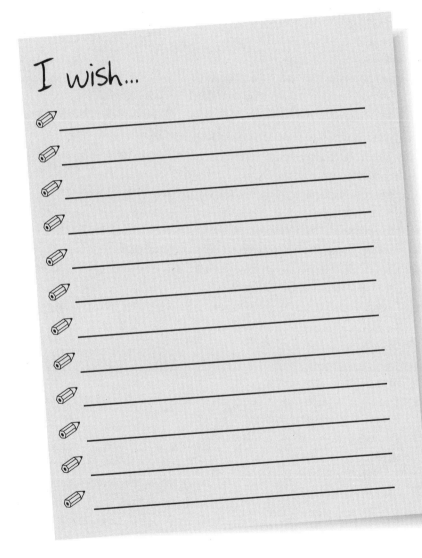

I wish...

Survivors say...

What do you wish someone would have said or done during your cancer?

- Emotional support at home. *Diana, 46, lung*
- "This is not the end of the world." *Jim, 50, thyroid*
- About not using my arm for heavy lifting. *Rosalie, 80, breast*
- Destroy all side effect information you receive prior to your chemotherapy. *Mary, 52, breast*
- Minister never called or came by. *Dorothy, 70, breast*
- Come see me. Don't run away. *Robert, 70, lung*
- Be more supportive and considerate of my emotions. *L, 58, breast*
- A person tried to make me feel guilty about not working during my time on chemo. *Mary, 62, breast*
- More humor in their conversations. *Murray, 64, lymphoma*
- I was lucky. I had great support! *Theresa, 49, breast*
- To talk or call my wife. Some people probably didn't know what to do, so they did nothing. Just call the spouse. *Bill, 64, throat, tongue*
- Take some time off. *Joseph, 25, Hodgkin's lymphoma*
- I know people handle things differently, but it hurt when people I worked with or knew never even said anything such as, "I'm sorry to hear you have to go through this." *Barbara, 48, breast*
- "I know someone who is a survivor of this type of cancer, let me have you meet with them." *Norma, 56, mesothelomia*
- They said I would lose my hair and have burns on my body following treatments. Neither was true! *Barb, 62, breast and thyroid*
- That it wasn't my fault. There is a lot of self blame. I always had mammograms and yearly checkups, but still felt guilty for missing it. *Noreen, 49, breast*

Communication between the sexes

Best-selling author John Gray's book *Men are From Mars, Women are From Venus* discusses the differences between the sexes. Widely accepted in general terms, Gray defines the differences in gender as it relates to issues related to physical, emotional, spiritual and sexual aspects of life.

There are some important gender differences we need to understand if we want to effectively communicate with our loved ones. Here are some typical differences:

▸ Women tend to process feelings externally while men process feelings internally

▸ Women tend to talk in a circular fashion to find their own answers, while men tend to reflect internally in a linear fashion as a means of finding solutions

▸ Men tend to attempt to "fix" problems, while women tend to talk through problems

▸ Women need to feel "cared for" while men need to feel "appreciated"

▸ Women want to feel respected and loved, while men want to feel trusted and valued

▸ Men see things from an analytical and logical viewpoint, while women see things from a feeling, intuitive and helping perspective

▸ Men tend to go into their "cave" when they try to figure out solutions, while women tend to want to talk about their concerns with others

▸ Men tend to feel relieved if they are left alone, while women hate to be left alone

▸ Men have to have proof that something is true, while women can believe it to be true

▸ Men offer solutions, while women need to find their own way

▸ Men tend to shut down their feelings, while women need to explore their emotions

- Men tend to use anger to avoid hurt and fear, while women use worry and fear to avoid anger
- Men speak to make a point, while women speak to discover and communicate

Why is it important to know these things? We need to know because men and women process things differently. You may think you are "communicating" with the opposite sex, but they may not really be hearing or understanding what's important to you. By knowing gender differences, you can learn to communicate more effectively with your loved one in a voice that the other gender can actually hear!

Jumpstart a conversation

- Avoid "yes" and "no" questions
- Concentrate on "how" and "why" questions
- Ask a question that will automatically lead to another
- Incorporate "I" statements as much as possible to personalize the conversation
- Don't ask, "Did you have a good day?" Say, "Tell me how your day has been. What did you do specifically? Why was it a good (bad) day?"
- Don't just ask, "What can I do for you?" Instead try, "Would it be all right if I do (something specific)?" or "I'd like to do (something specific)."
- Encourage responses with "Tell me how you feel about ..."
- Possible conversation topics:
    - children, grandchildren
    - sports
    - movies, other entertainment
    - upcoming events
    - hobbies
    - something funny
    - local or national news
    - family history
    - new and unusual products in the marketplace
- If you're really brave: politics and religion.
- And thank goodness there's always the weather!

While in search of positives, reality adds much reflection

Reflecting on the past, Ellyn rests her hand against the cap covering her bald head.

In the fall of 1997, she thought she was just experiencing some stomach problems, which persisted until she finally went to her physician. Though eventually diagnosed as an ovarian cyst, it was actually ovarian cancer. It was hoped that it was all caught in surgery shortly after Thanksgiving.

"I thought, 'that's good.' There was a 25 percent chance I'd get it again, but 75 percent I wouldn't. Unfortunately, I was the 25 percent." She laughs and shakes her head. During that time, her oldest son was getting married, and her future daughter-in-law's mother also had cancer.

Two years later, "I was in great shape. I worked every day. My life went on. I was happy, I knew I was going to beat this. I had friends and family, and everybody was so happy."

But it came back. However, she wouldn't let it deter her from fulfilling a long-time dream to visit Israel.

Ellyn beat it again and faithfully visited the doctor every two to three months. However, it returned a third time two years later when her daughter was getting married. Again, she won that battle.

In the fall of 2004, she thought she had a bad sinus infection and was on medication for many weeks until she worsened. The stunning diagnosis was a rare occurrence of ovarian cancer migrating to her brain. Chemo wouldn't help this time. "I had slipped through the cracks again. This could happen. That's why I want people to know this could happen to anyone." She had always had regular pap smears, though that's not an indicator of ovarian cancer.

She was very positive the first time, vowing to beat it as she continued to work every day. "I just pretended it didn't happen."

How did she do that?

"I guess with the coping skills I have. I have the tendency to take things in my head and then I work them through, see what I can do and see how I change things for the better. Always positive." She had always been that way, a valuable skill she applied to her career as a teacher. She researched everything she could find on ovarian cancer and consulted a myriad of physicians.

Family and friends assisted her in every way. Yet, the first time, she found herself comforting them, "telling them everything was okay, I was okay ... I put on a very, very courageous face ... not letting on how scared I was."

How did she handle those fears? By talking to a counselor and a rabbi, and keeping a journal for a year and a half. "One part in the journal was lots of love and positive, and one part was very black ... I couldn't handle telling them how bad it was, how scared I was, all these things happening to me. I didn't know what to do about them. I would just write it all down." She acknowledges that it took her a long time to express those fears aloud to her family. "They no longer have to wait for me to say, 'I'm scared.' I will say it now."

How did she get past that fear?

The counselor helped her realize who is more important and gave her the courage to get past that fear. " 'You've got to get it out. They need to know.' "

What were those initial fears?

"Fear of death ... not being able to finish my family's life, not being able to see my family grow up, my grand-children not knowing me, my family forgetting me."

> **Lesson #1**
> It's okay to talk about how scared you are

She admits that she has not coped with all those emotions yet.

"I cry a lot. I don't know ... I need to talk to more people about how to do this. I'm not sure how you cope with these feelings."

What lessons has she learned along the way?

"Pretending it isn't me. It was somebody else and it's going away. It went away before, it will go away again. By the fourth time, however, that wasn't there anymore." The reality saturates her voice. Yes, the first time shock, the second time, "I can do it again"; third time, "I guess I can do it again." This fourth time? "How the hell am I ever going to get through this again?"

"People realized it was coming back, but that I beat it before, I'm going to beat it again ... People would say to me, 'You're so coura-geous.' 'No, not really.' " She laughs.

How does she define courage compared to seven years earlier?

Herein lies the longest pause of the conversation.

"I'm not sure I have courage. I think the old courage is gone. It's hard for me to say. I'm certainly not putting on a happy face for everyone anymore. I can't do that. It's more important for me to let some of this out because they want to know. I'll do the best I can."

She credits her close friend Evelyn Vogel for helping start "Ellyn's Whisper," an educational organization to spread awareness about this silent cancer, ovarian. "If I have to go through it, someone should know about it. It makes it easier for them. You have to be your own advocate."

Ellyn says her battle against cancer has been a difficult emotional journey for her and her family. Her husband, daughter and two sons have responded in different ways. She smiles with a maternal knowledge of how her children find it difficult to accept that their mother could be dying, how they brush it off with a positive, "No, Mom, please, you're going to be fine," when she discusses what the future may bring.

Lesson #2
Cancer is a tough emotional battle for everyone

She faced her grim prognosis and opted for hospice care in early 2005. When asked how she came to grips with that, she says her faith is "up and down," how God is there for her at times and other times absent. Her rabbi told her that if she's angry at God, then there has to be one, though she did tell one doctor there was no God. She shakes her head at the rational, yet conflicting emotions.

When asked if she was still cautious with vocalizing her thoughts because she doesn't want to hurt anyone's feelings, she nods. However, she's getting better about speaking up, she says with a smile.

Coping with cancer and the limitations it has placed on her remain an ongoing frustration. It drives this once-independent woman crazy needing someone all the time because she can't make dinner, can't get out of chair, can't go to the bathroom by herself, and can't even shop or clean.

"Makes me nuts." She sighs under the cap atop her bald head. "I try to listen to people talking so I can get my mind focused. I love to read, but I can't read, and that makes me really irritated. I can't go on the computer. Sometimes I want to take everything in the house and smash it to smithereens."

The long pause prompts the inevitable question, "Have you smashed anything?" Once, she did bash something around the house and another time threw a puzzle off the table. "I guess it helped." It's suggested that she get some cheap dishes to fling, an image that generates a refreshing laugh.

Being with her family has been her primary motivation in fighting cancer's seemingly endless onslaught. Her biggest goal is welcoming her first grandchild in the spring of 2005. That news alone has given her a new and mighty arsenal as she and her daughter talk about sonograms and literally watch this new life develop. Ellyn giggles as she revisits those exciting moments so far.

While the future brings excitement, it also prompts reflection.

"Certain things don't mean much to me. At one point if my house were a mess, I would never allow anyone to come in. Now I don't care. As long as they come in, it's just fine." Even when her daughter brings her dog over on the new carpet, Ellyn doesn't care. "People and friendship and family and love are the most important things. People don't think ... they take life for granted. Things going along, happy, day by day."

However, cancer has been a gradual acceptance on her part.

"By the fourth time, it hit me in the head ... literally."

She wants her life lessons to educate others. Ellyn's Whisper is one way.

"What Evelyn did for me ... I cannot tell you how wonderful that was. It was exactly what I wanted, and she did it." Her tears start. "There are certain people I know I can talk to, I can say certain things to."

Ellyn's message about communicating with loved ones and friends simply echoes one component of this journey we call life, a more hazardous passage when cancer detours our path. It's not easy to convey the whirlwind of emotions.

Lesson #3
People, friendship, family and love are the most important things

"They're trying to help me get through this part. They're pushing on my legacy to help other people. It's not bad that I cry. They can cry with me, too."

Humor helps her cope as she's learned to laugh at herself and her lack of hair. However, she wasn't always able to do that because she was extremely shy for many years. Cancer changed that. "I'm going to do my own thing ... to a certain extent." She laughs again.

She can't deny that there are days when she admits she's tired and literally wants to "give up." She listens to family and friends' positive and encouraging words, but there are certain truths only she can absorb and comprehend.

Ellyn knows that the human spirit can bounce back, hers specifically, after being broken down fighting so many battles. However, if her present treatment doesn't work, she won't go back for chemo. "I'm not going to put myself through it," the extra pain if there's no hope, though she's fought it with every cell of her weakened body. At this particular moment, she admits she had not found peace and acceptance yet. "I need to talk to a few more people."

Part of her "speaking" has been writing letters to relatives and loved ones. The act of putting pen to paper has been therapeutic as she brings to life what she wants to say to each of them. She's telling them how much she loves them, how each are special to her, how wonderful each have been to her, how each have had a special place in her heart. For her three children, "How much I love them, which I always tell them anyway. Whenever I say goodbye, I always say, 'I love you.' How when they were little, all the things I did for them because I loved them, some of the funny things that happened. My husband, the same thing."

However, she admits, "I can't be courageous on everything," as she notes the anger and again that desire to smash things at times. Is that just part of being human? "I'm trying," she adds, chuckling. And part of being human is that bond with those she loves and how important their actions, words and presence have been every minute.

"As long as you're here with me, I don't care. I might be sleeping. But you're sitting with me, being with me. You thought enough of me to be here. There is nothing you can really say because you can't change anything, no matter what you do. You'd like to try, but there's nothing you can do."

Lesson #4
Find the way you're most comfortable with to communicate

Her friends have truly responded.

"I'm amazed I have this many friends. I just don't know where they're coming from. It makes me feel wonderful. It's sort of sad, but I think about how I'm going to have a funeral one day, as we all are. I'm going to have a lot of people, which is a very sad thought, but there are a lot of people who thought a lot of me. I'm amazed. I can't get that in my head that I've done something for them that they're doing so much for me."

What does she wish others would have done or said?

"That's really hard. I don't know. I want them to accept what could possibly happen to me. Not that I'm giving up, but that they understand and that my life on this earth could be much shorter than we all wanted it to be."

But isn't that her comforting them?

She laughs at the irony.

"I know. I just can't get that out of my head." She hesitated telling people in the beginning. "I had to do what I had to do, write those journals, write some things that are pretty horrible." She's gone back and read them. Expressing her emotions did help her tremendously. "I felt so much better to get it down. Sometimes I'd read it over and over. I got it out, out of my mind."

Isn't that a lesson for anybody, for everybody?

"You can't keep these things in. You have to be able to express yourself." Is she more expressive than she used to be? "I say more than I used to say." It eases the emotional burden.

What does she recommend other people say to cancer patients?

Be supportive, make sure they're getting the treatment they need, that they're taking care of themselves. Cancer patients should be honest with their loved ones immediately. "Don't give up until the very, very last second if at all possible." To her, giving up implies you don't care. "I won't give up."

In the beginning, she says, act natural, life goes on, make it as normal as possible. She didn't want to go to support groups to listen to other people, though it was important for her to talk to somebody or jot those thoughts on paper. She doesn't let other people's expectations and worries derail her. She seeks the positive, yet is realistic.

Ellyn just wants to enjoy life.

Postscript: *Ellyn followed her own advice and didn't give up until the very last second of her life ... April 16, 2005, her 61st birthday, a month before the arrival of her first grandchild. She had been excited about this book and hoped that her insight could help others cope with the toll that cancer can exert on the survivor and loved ones. Ellyn's words and love will stir far more people than she could have ever imagined. She certainly changed our lives and reassured us of the importance of this book and life itself.*

Lesson #5
Don't let other people's expectations and worries derail you

Survivors say...

110

What advice would you give to help with the different emotional responses of friends and family?

▶ Do not dwell on the condition and keep a positive attitude. Offer support and follow up on support. *Ralph, 68, prostate*

▶ My friends were very positive. Stressed "you'll be okay." *Jude, 64, breast*

▶ Accept people as they are. *C, 79, breast*

▶ They'll calm down if you are hopeful. *Betty, 68, breast*

▶ Just tell them you want them to go on with their life as before. *Betty, 75, breast*

▶ Be real, open, honest and up front about everything. *Linda, 62, breast*

▶ I honestly don't have any. I myself had a hard time with this part. Everyone was different. *Robin, 46, breast*

▶ Several people I thought were friends immediately dropped out of my life. I decided they were too afraid to stay, and I concentrated on everyone who did stay. *Karen, 62, breast*

> "If you don't know what to say, you can show support by listening, praying or just saying you're sorry this is happening to them." *Mary, 52, breast*

▶ Ask for prayers and let them respond as they see fit. If felt appropriate, inject a little humor. *Joseph, 80, bladder*

▶ Be firm, but willing to accept more than you can give. Learn to say no. *Judy, 69, colon*

- Everyone reacts and accepts differently. *Dorothy, 70, breast*
- Realize that they do not know what you feel unless they have been there. *Robert, 70, lung*
- Listen. You can't fix it. Show your true concern and compassion. Care for them. Pray, pray and pray. *L, 58, breast*
- Think in terms of recovery. *Kathy, 61, breast*
- Study how they can give positive support. *Mary, 62, breast*
- Let people respond to you. They need to, also. You need the emotional support, and they need to give it. *Mary Ann, 56, colon*
- Keep a good sense of being. *Murray, 64, lymphoma*
- If you don't know what to say, you can tell them just that you are thinking of them and will keep them in your thoughts and prayers. *Diane, 47, breast*
- We live in a time of medical advances. Support the fight. Give unconditional love. Let your emotions be known. *Gresha, 47, breast*
- Tell them not to give up on the person with cancer. *Rita, 58, breast*
- Some people won't understand your pain. *Bill, 64, throat and tongue*
- Let the person cry when they are sad. *Paula, 53, uterine and breast*
- My son talked about my breast cancer to friends and teachers, and my daughter told no one. *Barbara, 48, breast*
- Be prepared for remarks that are thoughtless. Don't be hurt by those who say nothing. *Helen, 72, lung*
- People love you and want to do the right thing. If they are struggling or awkward in responding, let them know you appreciate their caring. *Carolyn, 70, colon*
- Surround yourself with only caring, positive, upbeat people. Avoid those who are negative or depressing. *Lorraine, 48, breast*

"Express concern, but try not to be too emotional. The patient needs to be able to grieve, not to comfort someone else."
Joseph, 25, Hodgkin's lymphoma

111

▸ Keep in mind that everyone will respond in their own, unique way. As individuals, they will seek a manageable comfort level. Stay open-minded. There is no built-in guidebook for this. *Jennifer, 42, breast*

▸ Tell them that positive responses and attitudes aid greatly in coping and healing. *Barb, 62, breast and thyroid*

▸ Treat me the same. Help me keep my family routine. *Noreen, 49, breast*

▸ During my year of surgery and treatments, my mom would often tell people that I was handling all of this much better than she was. It is probably harder for your family and friends to cope with this, because at least you are able to do something, while they are bystanders. *Melinda, 46, breast*

▸ Grin and bear it. Ask friends to drive you to treatments. But most turned me down because down deep they thought I would get sick in their car or they were too busy. Rely on cancer support people for rides. *Carol, 71, colon*

▸ We don't want them to pity us, just to give us empathy, not sympathy. *Vicki, 53, breast*

▸ Try to surround yourself with those who make you stronger. *Diane, 38, thyroid*

▸ Be realistic, optimistic and empathetic, yet convey at this time that *you* are the one primarily in need of focus. *Clair, 55, breast*

▸ Let them digest what they can when they can. *Cheryl, 48, rectal*

"People should not stop coming around just because they're afraid they don't know what to say to you." Lori, 39, melanoma

Hello, I'm here!

Dear

Hey, I just wanted to let you know that I'm still the same person I was before I was diagnosed with cancer. I have just a few new basic needs:

- Please don't whisper around me or talk as if I'm not here. My hearing works just fine.
- Please don't act like I'm dying. I'm working very hard to beat this, and I'm surviving right now!
- Please don't ignore my cancer and how I'm affected emotionally by it.
- Please don't focus only on my cancer. The other 99% of me is working just fine or just has some down days occasionally.
- Please don't forget me and the unique needs of my loved ones during this time.
- Please remember that I need your support and not your critique of my life decisions.
- Please remember that I may be scared at times. I know you will be, too, and that's OK!

Love,

Hey, we need to talk!

One of the harsh realities of cancer is that the world keeps revolving, never stopping for one event or one person. Responsibilities continue, bills must still be paid, duties must be fulfilled, household chores must be juggled or delegated.

When cancer strikes a family, the immediate response is and should be to address the medical needs of the patient. With this crisis come new questions and worries. Let's start with insurance:

▶ *What will our medical insurance cover? What's not covered?*

▶ *What has to be pre-approved or pre-certified?*

▶ *Is a second opinion covered or required by the insurance?*

▶ *What's our maximum lifetime coverage? What's our co-pay?*

▶ *Does the insurance limit where I can go or what doctors I see?*

▶ *Are there limits on prescriptions? Are generics an option?*

▶ *Do we have more than one source of insurance coverage?*

▶ *Do I qualify for home health care services?*

▶ *Disability insurance:* Are you eligible? For how long?

▶ *Life insurance:* What policies are in effect? Are the beneficiaries up-to-date?

▶ *Monthly bills:* Can payments be made automatically to avoid them being overdue? Do you need to establish a financial power-of-attorney to pay bills if hospitalized or incapacitated?

▶ *Credit cards, loans:* What arrangements need to be made to avoid extra finance charges? Have all obligations been accounted for?

▶ *Wills:* Have valid and current wills been drawn up?

▶ *Living wills and advanced directives:* Have these been prepared? Does the family know and understand my wishes?

▶ *Investments:* Is all pertinent information up-to-date?

▶ *Do spouses/significant others know the location of any and all financial information?*

▶ *Have parents informed adult children of these arrangements and where all information can be found?*

Checklist

How's my financial and legal health?

When was the last time I checked my medical insurance coverage? What's changed? _____

_____

What life insurance policies do I have? Who are the agents?

_____

_____

_____

Do I have disability or long-term care insurance privately or through work? What are the requirements and limits? _____

_____

Is my spouse/significant other aware of where all policies and paperwork can be found? Where are they? _____

_____

_____

_____

Do we have a safety deposit box? Where is it located and who has a key? _____

_____

If I have adult children or parents, are they aware of where paper-work and information can be found if I need their assistance, especially if they live out of town? How will I inform them? _____

116 _____

Do I have a close friend or relative who can assist with some of these details? _____

_____

Do I have a valid and up-to-date will? If so, where is it and who was the attorney? _____

_____

What sources of income do I have in the event I'm off work? Disability? Insurance? Investments? _____

_____

_____

What's the status of all my investments? When was the last time those were evaluated? Who's the financial advisor? Do I have an accurate picture of my net worth, liabilities and assets?

_____

_____

_____

Have I set up durable power-of-attorney for all legal decisions in case I am incapacitated? If so, who is that? If not, who should it be?

_____

_____

Do I have a living will and/or advanced directive that will outline my wishes in case I am incapacitated? Do I have copies I can take everywhere I need to go? Are my loved ones aware of my wishes?

_____

_____ 117

_____

Have I completed funeral pre-planning? If yes, are my loved ones aware of this? What funeral home or director? Have my wishes changed since I made those arrangements? If yes, who should I contact? If I have selected cremation, are my loved ones aware of this?

_____

_____

_____

_____

_____

Do my loved ones understand and have they accepted my decisions on all matters related to death? _____

_____

_____

_____

_____

_____

_____

_____

_____

Making sense of $$$

▸ I wish we would have checked out finances better and what I should do with the insurance. But what he did say was everything I needed to hear. *Colleen, 60, husband, colon*

▸ Wish I had forced him to talk to me about what I needed to do financial-wise since I had no knowledge of bill paying or calling for repairs. Needed a book on how to budget, take or keep a list for taxes and how to handle money and bills, and call for help when needed rather than take physical chances. *Bertha, 84, husband, prostate*

▸ (Wished had) learned more about finances earlier. *Virginia, 66, husband, colon; mother-in-law, colon*

▸ One dear friend took care of my bills, sent them to Medicare and my health insurance company. Kept all bills up to date. I was too ill to do so. *Alveretta, 85, ovarian*

▸ I took over everything I could. He was upset by some of it, like paying his bills and taking care of his mail, but he was glad not to have to worry about lots of things since he usually felt awful. *Monica, 35, husband, pancreatic*

▸ Our office collected money. We also gave gas cards and phone cards for those long trips to cancer clinics. We bought non-perishable food to help with keeping the family fed. *Diane, 38, friend/co-worker, breast*

▸ I assumed tasks that had been his domain. *Edith, 65, husband, melanoma*

"He liked to be in charge. That changed when he was too sick to make decisions." *Mary, 52, husband, kidney*

Offering

assistance

"What we have done for ourselves alone dies with us; what we have done for others and the world remains and is immortal." Albert Pike

Asking for help is not always easy

120

Many times significant others have difficulty knowing what they can do to assist their loved one. As a result, they end up feeling helpless.

There are many things you can do to help. We've tried to break these down into tasks or things that you can do physically, and have created a list of emotional ways in which you can support your loved one.

Remember, you may not be asked for your assistance … in fact, our research indicates that many survivors won't ask but later feel hurt or resentful. Locked in their own world, many survivors tell us they have difficulty reaching out for help, because they have always been the one to help others. They tell us they just didn't have the skills to know how to ask for help without feeling guilty.

It's important for you to know that our research indicates most of our significant others did not ask what they could do; they just waited for the survivor to tell them. We believe this puts additional pressure on your survivor and just makes both parties feel helpless and in some ways very hopeless.

We know you aren't a mind reader, but it goes without saying, it never hurts to ask what would be most helpful during this time period. Trust us, they may not tell you, but it doesn't hurt to just ask. Give your loved one a copy of these suggestions and have them circle the items that would be of help!

The following are some of the most common suggestions from survivors and caretakers concerning some physical tasks you can do to assist your loved one:

- Come home during the day to visit
- Drive them to appointments with physician
- Give medical assistance
- Tell them "I love you"
- Drive them to treatments and wait with them
- Hold the survivor's hand during chemotherapy
- Make phone calls during the day, just to say hello

- Advocate for the survivor with physicians and health care workers
- Help with the cooking
- Help maintain normality in the survivor's life
- Be there to do anything
- Help the survivor take a bath
- Help with bathroom duty
- Help the survivor gather information or research on treatment, types of cancers, successful options, etc.
- Keep the environment light and cheerful
- Provide hugs
- Encourage the survivor to exercise and eat nutritionally
- Cry with the survivor
- Help change dressings
- Take the survivor on little tours or errands to keep their mind off the diagnosis
- Read books of inspiration to the survivor
- Take the survivor for little special food "treats"
- Stay with the survivor in the hospital
- Take the survivor to lunch
- Provide a sense of stability, financial support, and protection from the outside world when they feel overwhelmed
- Go for a short walk together

- Initiate talks about treatment options
- Write encouraging notes, cards or send e-mails
- Move in with survivor, when not living together
- Encourage the survivor to solicit a second opinion
- Make appointments for the survivor
- Arrange for someone to come in and cut and style your survivor's hair
- Research hospice care
- Take over daily chores
- Hire a cleaning person to help with the home
- Hire a babysitter or nanny to help with the children
- Keep a daily diary of the survivor's progress for the physician appointments
- Keep a list of questions to be asked of the hospital, physician and oncologist
- Arrange for a massage therapist appointment with a provider who has special training related to cancer patients

121

Allow the survivor the opportunity to make their own choices and decisions

122

- Research best oncologists and hospitals
- Administer medication
- Maintain a sexual relationship
- Organize medication in pill boxes according to daily requirements
- Give them a backrub
- Give the survivor a foot and hand massage with lotion
- Bring home small gifts
- Help them with "final arrangements" and preparations for death
- Arrange to take them out to dinner with friends
- Take care of the mail and bills
- Fluff pillows for the survivor in bed
- Help them dress
- Take care of the pets
- Help feed the survivor when needed
- Offer to shave your head in support of your survivor
- Help administer shots
- Draw a bubble bath for them to relax
- Listen to music together
- Practice meditation or breathing exercises together
- Do stretching exercises together
- Do yoga together
- Look at the stars

Talk about who influenced or mentored your life

- Share stories about positive experiences in your lives
- Plant flowers together
- Tell jokes and bring laughter into their life
- Talk about things for which you are "grateful"
- Attend a sports event or watch it together on television
- Read to your loved one
- Go to the park and play on the swings
- Go to a play, a movie or a concert
- Draw a picture together
- Lay on a blanket in the grass and imagine figures in the clouds
- Make a special meal together
- Take a car ride to a special place
- Have a picnic in the park
- Talk about your dreams for the future
- Make snow angels
- Talk about childhood experiences or funny stories in your past

- Take a ride and look at the fall foliage
- Write funny poems or limericks together
- Watch funny movies together like the Marx Brothers or WC Fields
- Go outside and blow bubbles
- Talk about what you love about each other
- Make floral arrangements from flowers in the yard
- Talk about your successes
- Go get facials together
- Paint a color by numbers picture together
- Share special hugs
- Spend time putting a puzzle together

- Go for a ride in a convertible
- Ride through the drive-thru in your pajamas
- Get a box of 64 crayons and color together
- Play card games like Crazy Eights, War, or double solitaire
- Make chocolate milk shakes or banana splits together
- Create a collage of pictures of those who are important to your loved one
- Go to the pet shop and play with the puppies
- Buy new sheets or pajamas
- Bring fuzzy slippers for chemo or home

123

Top responses

- Significant other was 'just there'
- Assisted with daily tasks
- Offered to be there to do any task
- Significant other says 'I love you'
- Drive to medical appointments

Survivors say...

What did your friends do or say to assist you?

▶ Since I am a very private person, it never occurred to me to tell friends and family that I had cancer and a mastectomy. To this day, very few people know of this. No, I was not in denial. How can a person deny a mastectomy and lymphoma and all that with surgery? *N, 80, breast*

▶ Unconditional acceptance. *Rosalie, 80, breast*

▶ Stayed with me. Told me that I can get better. *Karen, 51, lung*

▶ Most didn't know what to do. A few were very open and sharing. Some seemed to prepare for separation. *Robert, 70, lung*

▶ One took me to radiation once. Others always asked and let me know they care, especially my pastor. *C, 79, breast*

▶ Everything possible. Couldn't have made it without their help and prayers. *Dorothy, 70, breast*

▶ Gave me cards and books that were helpful and at the same time humorous. Visited me in the hospital. And most of all, hugs! *Elaine, 72, leukemia*

▶ Not much. People don't understand if they haven't been through it. *Donna, 72, colon*

▶ Cards, flowers, some phone calls. Didn't really want to talk much. Lots of prayer chains. *Maria, 61, breast*

▶ Encouraged me, told how well I was doing. Listened! *Theresa, 49, breast*

▶ My friends didn't want to talk about it. *Marilyn, 72, breast*

▶ Most said they were sorry for me. Some offered to drive me to my treatments or other assistance. *Murray, 64, lymphoma*

▶ They just wanted to know how I was doing and gave encouragement. They did not dwell on condition. *Ralph, 68, prostate*

▶ Ignored it. *J, 81, breast*

- Food, cards, flowers, faith, ongoing caring, keeping in touch, tried not to overkill. *Judy, 69, colon*

- Talked and joked with me. *Noor, 56, breast*

- They didn't know. *G, 81, uterine*

- I didn't tell anyone until after surgery. *Robin, 46, breast*

- They sent inspirational cards and dropped by or called pretty often to cheer me up. I received two phone cards. One cleaned my fridge, one took me to a healing mass, one paid to have my house cleaned. *Mary Ann, 56, colon*

- They encouraged me and supported me in going out socially with them when I felt better. *Mary, 62, breast*

- Occasional visits. One friend offered to shave her head and smoke marijuana with me! I declined! *Gresha, 47, breast*

- Certain ones were good. Others not. I felt better with people being concerned about my wife. *Bill, 64, throat and tongue*

- I received so many cards, phone calls and flowers at the beginning. During the treatment process, I became pretty isolated, and my friends were always there to listen even when I didn't want to be here. *Paula, 53, uterine and breast*

- Accepted me and my decisions and supported me. Provided emotional and humorous support, not to mention months of meals. *Judy, 56, breast*

- Prayed. Took me to lunch. Stayed upbeat. *Sandy, 58, breast*

- They called me and told me of their friends who had gotten through this. *Martha, 51, breast*

> "My co-workers provided two meals per week on the weeks I had chemotherapy (six months). My friend took reflexology and worked on me two to three times a month."
> Mary, 52, breast

- Hang in there. You can beat this. I also was off work eight months and had the support of fellow workers. *Okdoke, 67, uterine*

▸ Presented a very sincere concern for me. *Janet, 65, breast*

▸ A couple of them had been through the same surgery, mastectomy, and shared their experiences with me. *Julie, 61, breast*

▸ They visited me, sent me little packages, e-mailed, called. Some brought lunch, and we ate at the house or went out when I felt better. *Carolyn, 70, colon*

▸ For the most part by treating me as they always had. *Jennifer, 42, breast*

▸ All of my wonderful friends listened with me, cried with me, laughed with me, and were always willing to help me. *Norma, 56, mesothelomia*

▸ At first, they felt awkward, afraid to talk about it, and now they have loosened up and are even joking about the situation to lighten the matter. *Sara, 35, lung*

▸ My friends were a huge blessing. The most important thing they did was consistently getting together to pray. Lots of encouragement and truly caring about me and my family. They loved and provided for my children's emotional needs, letting them cry when they needed to, promising to be there. *Noreen, 49, breast*

▸ They brought my lunch, stayed with me. *Carol, 71, colon*

▸ I felt most were afraid to talk about it, and my bosses did not realize some things that I felt they would know, and so I was afraid to ask for help. *Barbara, 61, breast*

▸ My co-workers were always there for me with positive words of encouragement. A long-time friend from school days bought me my first bandanna, and we shared many tears together. *Vicki, 53, breast*

▸ I had a tracheostomy and was non-verbal, so my friends were awesome visiting and not expecting me to talk, which was difficult physically but also emotionally. They also cooked, took care of my kids, and had a fundraiser to help with costs. *Diane, 38, thyroid*

▸ I love you, ditto, ditto, ditto. Everyone was so willing to help my son and make sure he still had a fun life. *Cheryl, 48, rectal*

Please, please 'bother' me!

A cancer patient doesn't feel well for a couple of days but says nothing until the situation becomes a medical emergency.

"I didn't want to bother anyone."

A survivor hurts themselves while doing something beyond their physical capability early in their recuperation.

"I didn't want to bother anyone."

Another survivor keeps their fears to themselves and refuses to talk about them until they've worked themselves into a depressed state. The emotional response begins to affect their physical recovery.

"I didn't want to bother anyone."

Virtually everybody wants to be able to take care of themselves, to be independent, to be self-reliant. They hate it when they have to depend on others — loved ones, friends and strangers — for specialized assistance or even the most basic of needs. These patients may think they're making life easier on everyone around by not "bothering" them, but in reality, they may make what would have been a simple response into a more serious one that may become life-threatening or financially costly.

Yes, caregivers and family members will become physically fatigued and emotionally exhausted while caring for anyone with a serious illness, but most want to be *"bothered"* because offering assistance is a way for them to deal emotionally with the entire situation. As many of our survey respondents noted, cancer takes a toll on everyone, yet it can be a precious bonding experience. Caregivers feel helpless sitting or standing around *"doing nothing."*

That's why our loved ones and friends have earned that special place in our lives and our hearts, because of the powerful relationship that has been established by birth or by a chance meeting. That bond should speak for itself, *"I'm here for you when you need me."* Just like the oft-quoted message, *"Friends don't let friends drive drunk,"* in cancer it should be, *"Friends don't let friends go through this alone."*

Remember, you'd do the same for them.

Consider this very powerful observation from a survivor:

Offering to help someone makes them feel like a burden or unable to care for themselves. It's the doing that really helps. Subtle encouragement and persistent comfort, physical and emotional, is nice. Touch is nice in order to reassure the person isn't diseased. A hug or even friendly patting.

You are not a burden!

128

"All of us tried to be there so he wouldn't have to ask for help. It's not easy to ask, so we made sure we were just 'there.'" Mary, 42, father, lung

"I arranged my schedule to be with my parents for as many office visits and chemo treatments as possible. We all had to be very proactive because my parents won't ask for help." Carlene, 51, mother, breast

"If I had not heard from her for a week, I would call or stop by to see her. Got her help as the disease progressed. She did not want her friends cleaning or cooking for her and family." Mary, 63, best friend, breast

Loved ones say...

In what ways do you believe you were able to assist the patient physically and emotionally?

▶ Physically, we are just entering our journey, so we'll see. Emotionally, I let him ask the questions that were important to him and let him talk about his fears. *Laura, 44, father, prostate*

▶ I am a survivor. Find humor in situations. *Patricia, 64, husband, larynx*

▶ I was there every day from the first day to his last day on earth. *L, fiancee, kidney*

▶ We held each other more often. I helped with his treatments. We prayed the rosary together. *Colleen, 60, husband, colon*

▶ Helped get home health equipment when it was needed. Never felt I helped emotionally. *Julie, 51, father, lung*

▶ He ate what I asked him to eat and was active as he could be. A smile was always there. *Marianne, 71, husband, large cell lymphoma*

▶ I'd overcome breast cancer 12 years earlier so was somewhat of a role model for "it can be overcome." There is life with and after cancer. *Judith, 70, husband, colon*

▶ I wasn't helpful because of my own insecurities. *Bette, 57, husband, melanoma*

▶ By just being there. My sister said that she did not realize how much love was around her. *Rosemary, 66, sister, ovarian*

▶ I did many personal physical things as his energy decreased. Offered unconditional love. *Barbara, 66, husband, larynx*

▶ Let him know that we were there for him, as he has always been there for us. *Mary, 42, father, lung*

▶ Even though he was much bigger than I was, I would pull him up from the chair and lockstep him to the bathroom or table. Always assured him it was okay. *Bertha, 84, husband, prostate*

130

- I tried to use humor and not envision a lifetime of living with a handicapped person. *Pat, 57, husband, brain*

- I was able to be there with her and act as her advocate when visiting with healthcare providers. She also knew she could tell me anything. *Carlene, 51, mother, breast*

- Kept her as comfortable as possible, changed her dressings, took care of her bodily needs, took her out as long as she was able. *Annamarie, 62, daughter, NA*

- Gave him manicures, pedicures, back rubs. Physical care when his strength failed. Just sat with him. *Shirley, 66, brother, lung*

- Physically I was able to help Mom to sit still and not cause herself to tire so quickly. Emotionally I was there. *Rue, 29, mother, breast*

- I was there to listen, sometimes to the point where I didn't want to hear about cancer. He became somewhat obsessed talking about it. *Patti, 52, husband, renal cell cancer*

- I am always there for her and I'm always positive with her. I would (and still do) tell her many times a day that I love her. *Randy, 46, wife, breast*

- I may not have understood everything emotionally, but I was there. *Dan, 44, wife, breast*

"He told me I was the one person he trusted completely to be there for him." Linda, 62, husband, colon

- I always supported his decisions. I never pushed him into treatment and never really said anything against his decisions. *Lisa, 40, husband, brain*

- Neither mastectomy or hysterectomy has affected our sex life or love relationship. *Robert, 53, wife, breast and uterine*

- Much of the time I was her primary caregiver. I tried to make sure all meds were taken on time and properly. I was her "cheerleader" but also respected all of her decisions. *Mark, 45, wife, breast*

- We never know what effect we have. Her determination kept us all upbeat. *Joan, 69, niece, lymphoma*

Loved ones say...

Did you offer specific assistance without being asked? If so, what? Or did you wait for the patient to ask?

Physical

▶ I came for his surgery, treatments and last weeks until death in February 1986. I didn't wait to be asked. He wanted me there. *C, 63, father, esophageal and liver*

▶ I did her laundry a couple of times each week. We took food and did a "group housecleaning." Took her shopping, hair appointments, car trips. I did not wait for her to ask. *Sharon, 65, friend, breast*

▶ We talked about best approaches (medical, alternative therapies, support groups, nutrition) together and decided on direction. *Paul, 53, wife, breast*

▶ I called more, and we saw each other at work. She picked different friends for different stages of her treatment. One helped shave her head. I gave her moral support as she gave herself shots daily until she got a handle on it. *Susan, 49, best friend, lymphoma*

▶ Get a pad and pencil. *Patricia, 64, husband, larynx*

▶ Household chores, cooking, driving to chemo and doctor. *Doug, 57, wife, breast*

▶ I took care of him in every way I could 24 hours a day. *L, fiancee, kidney*

▶ I arranged for her to be in a very comfortable setting. *Rosemary, 66, sister, ovarian*

▶ Yes, I stayed with her (moved in with her) so she would not be alone and was able to remain at home until her death two months later. *Tracy, 47, mother, lung*

▶ I was always by his side, anticipated thirst or hunger, helped him get to the bathroom and dress. *Bertha, 84, husband, prostate*

▸ I stayed with him in the hospital after his surgery for six days because he wanted me there. *Linda, 62, husband, colon*

▸ I offered information since I am a nurse, but tried to avoid too much information. Offered to go to appointments with him but avoided pushing. Respected his need for independence. *Laura, 44, father, prostate*

▸ Sometimes I was overly concerned about her ability to do normal tasks. *Annamarie, 62, daughter, NA*

▸ I did what I could to make him comfortable. For example, I made him a pillow to rest his head on the floor when he stretched out. *Abbie, 51, father, leukemia*

▸ I brought her to our home for the first and second days following surgery as she lives alone. Prepared food for her, checked on her after she went home. Took her to doctor appointments. *N, 68, friend, breast*

▸ There were times when I waited for her to ask. I lotioned her feet and hands, sat with her, tried to be positive. Not enough, looking back now. *Kathleen, 24, mother, breast*

"I waited for her to let me know. Sometimes she felt like people didn't think she could do things for herself at times. She doesn't like that, so I would let her tell me when she needs some things or someone to talk to." Barb, 44, best friend, non-Hodgkins lymphoma

Emotional assistance as essential as physical aid

It's obvious that survivors need assistance with physical tasks, but what many forget is the importance of meeting emotional needs. In fact, attending to our emotional needs may be more important to the well-being of the survivor than physical tasks at times. There is nothing more essential than knowing that you are loved, nurtured, cared for and heard.

Significant others can offer emotional support in many ways. The following is a list of emotional support ideas that are essential to our survivors:

▶ *Tell the survivor "you can beat this."* Have a positive outlook. This may not seem that important, but the survivor may look to you when they are scared, tired, or fearful. Positive affirmations are a very powerful element in recovery.

▶ *Provide encouragement and emotional support.* Our survivors need to have cheerleaders.

▶ *Just be there to "listen."* You don't need to give advice or "fix it," just be there with an open heart to listen.

▶ *Act as though nothing related to the cancer is embarrassing.* Remember that there are medical situations in which the survivor feels fearful that you will leave or will not be able to continue to see them in the same way. Many of our survivors feel fearful they will not be loved if they have a mastectomy, lose their hair or gain weight.

▶ *Show your love through your supportive smiles and acceptance.* These may seem simple, but your love means so much.

▶ *Accept the diagnosis and be supportive, even when it is difficult.*

▶ *Stress that "we are in this together" so the survivor does not feel alone.* Remind your survivor that they've faced adversity in the past, and they can make it through this together.

▶ *Assist by focusing on "today" versus focusing on the future.* Sometimes it is difficult to chase away stay fear and negative thoughts, but help your loved one see the positives of today and the importance of hope.

▶ *Give them unconditional love and acceptance.* This may seem simple, but many survivors are worried about abandonment and poor choices.

▶ *Treat them with respect, versus treating them like a victim, or as if they are fragile.* Your loved one needs to feel like you believe in them and their powers of perseverance.

134

▶ *Assist your survivor's emotional well being by reminding them they are courageous and strong.*

▶ *Just "be there" for the survivor.* This is the most important asset to many survivors.

▶ *Tell the survivor they are beautiful or handsome, no matter what occurs.*

▶ *Listen, listen, listen.* Open your heart and be willing to hear what your loved one has to say. You may be the only person they can tell about their fears of death or medical concerns.

▶ *Give reassurances and build their confidence in their own abilities to "beat" the disease.*

Top responses

✐ Maintain positive outlook
✐ Provide encouragement and emotional support
✐ Show and say 'I love you'
✐ Just listen
✐ Be compassionate and loving

Loved ones say...

Did you offer specific assistance without being asked?
If so, what? Or did you wait for the patient to ask?

Emotional

▸ My dad was a very private man. We only discussed doctor appointments and outcomes. Kept his daily living as normal as possible. No sitting and discussing this problem. *Georgia, 48, father, lung*

▸ Tried to get her husband to break his denial. *P, 66, sister-in-law, lung and bone*

▸ We read each other pretty well. *Fred, 63, wife, breast*

▸ Yes, offered to stay with him in the hospital. (He was very claustrophobic and fearful.) Also offered to come home with him for his death. Took him out occasionally. *Shirley, 66, brother, lung*

▸ I'd usually let him ask. If I tried to do some things, he'd get cranky and tell me he was able to do it. *Patti, 52, husband, RCC*

▸ I tried to help without making her feel helpless. *John, 69, wife, breast*

▸ Followed patient's lead to maintain professionalism. Was there a lot to talk or go to lunch initially. Then patient drew on other resources and was able to turn to family and routine more and more. *Ann, 51, friend, brain*

▸ We were going through difficult times. It took the focus off our relationship problems and put our focus on survival and helping her get through this. *Dan, 44, wife, breast*

▸ Offered support when being asked and offered it often. If you wait for people to call you and ask for help, they probably won't. *Pam, friend, breast and lung*

▸ I tried to anticipate what she would need so she could concentrate on one thing, getting well. *Chuck, 61, wife, rectal*

▶ I tried to pick up the slack knowing she would be unable to do what she had been doing. I would tell her often that she had only one job, take care of herself and get better. *Mark, 45, wife, breast*

▶ I always let him know that I would do whatever he needed. I tried not to smother him. I let him take care of himself until he absolutely couldn't. He knew his limitations. I didn't. *Lisa, 40, husband, brain*

▶ I usually waited for my mom to ask for assistance. This was pretty selfish, but again, I was always trying to be just "normal without cancer," and this involved neglecting and denying my mom. *Maureen, 23, mother, breast*

▶ I tried to anticipate what needed to be done, but most of the time I had to ask. *David, 67, wife, breast*

"I'd go to work, and when I came home, I went to work. My jobs weren't done until everyone was in bed and asleep. I was a caregiver 24/7. Caregiving is a full-time job. It never ends. It has no holidays. You are working, nurturing, visiting, taking care of physical needs, taking care of medications, making sure medications are right, etc. You are in charge of medical care and you have to know how to do things. You just step up and do it. There is no room for embarrassment. You can't be timid, you just do things." *L, wife, breast*

Checklist

I need your physical assistance, please

❑ Sit with me

❑ Bring me flowers _____

❑ Bring me reading material

   ❑ Magazines _____

   ❑ Books _____

   ❑ Other _____

❑ Bring me a new journal _____

❑ Take me shopping

   ❑ Clothing _____

   ❑ Grocery _____

   ❑ Bookstore _____

❑ Pick up my medications _____

❑ Drive me to treatments _____

❑ Clean for me

   ❑ My bedroom _____

   ❑ My office _____

   ❑ Bathroom _____

   ❑ Kitchen _____

   ❑ Outside _____

over

Cancer: Here's how YOU can help ME cope & survive

❑ Take me to the movies

❑ Bring me some videos/DVDs

❑ _____

❑ _____

❑ Bring me some music

❑ _____

❑ _____

❑ Bring me some books

❑ _____

❑ _____

❑ Prepare something special to eat

❑ _____

❑ Take me out for a drive _____

❑ Take me to the library _____

❑ Help with the children

❑ Help them with their homework _____

❑ Help them with errands _____

❑ Talk to them _____

❑ Take the kids to dinner _____

❑ Babysit _____

❑ Take them to a movie, the park or playground

❑ Help with physical needs

❑ Bathing   ❑ Bathroom

❑ Change dressings   ❑ Medication

❑ _____

Checklist

I need your emotional support, please

☐ Sit with me

☐ Talk to me

☐ Listen to me

☐ Tell me a funny story

☐ Watch a movie with me

☐ Hug me

☐ Tell me what's going on in your life

☐ Help keep others informed about my health

☐ Bring me a stuffed animal to hold

☐ Read to me

☐ Send me cards

☐ Send me e-mail

☐ Treat me normally

☐ Cry with me

☐ Tell me you love me

☐ Be encouraging and positive

☐ Remind me that "I can make it"

☐ _____

☐ _____

Little things...

      Many times people don't know what they could or should bring to a survivor when they visit them at home or in the hospital. Here are some little gifts you can give someone who is diagnosed with cancer:

Food

Pajamas

Robe

Sweets

Powder

Lotions

Massage oils

Perfume

Scarves or hats

Journals

Inspirational books

CDs

Cards

Balloons

Coloring books and
  crayons

Magazines

Candles

Framed photos

Movies

Playing cards

Puzzles

Soft blankets

Pillows

Teddy bears

Cookies

Flowers

Plants

Hand-held games

Little gifts for
  their children

Comic books

Humorous books

Snack mix

Fruit bowls

Ice cream/yogurt

Shawls

Loved ones say...

Did you experience hurt feelings when the patient turned down or ignored your assistance? If yes, why?

▶ No, I respect my dad's ability to maintain control. He knows I am here and willing to do *anything*, but *he* gets to make those decisions. *Laura, 44, father, prostate*

▶ I think he felt that he was useless and wanted to make some of his own decisions. *Colleen, 60, husband, colon*

▶ Yes, somewhat felt pushed away. *Virginia, 66, husband, colon; mother-in-law, colon*

▶ My husband only took care of himself when a "pill" was prescribed, not when proper eating, exercise, etc. were recommended. So, yes, I'd get upset when he did not do those things to help himself. *Judith, 70, husband, colon*

▶ Sometimes. As I tried to offer nutritional food and his appetite decreased, I became discouraged. *Barbara, 66, husband, larynx*

▶ Yes, he wasn't his reasonable self, wouldn't follow doctor's instructions at my urging. *P, 62, husband, throat and neck*

▶ Sometimes he didn't like me "hovering." *Mary, 52, husband, kidney*

▶ I wanted to do more. Had to back off at times to allow them their independence. *Vera, 73, several relatives*

▶ Yes! He told others how wonderful I was, but to me complained of what he called mistakes. Very depressing. *Bertha, 84, husband, prostate*

▶ He didn't cooperate with exercise, eating, etc. But what hurt most was his unwillingness to share. *Linda, 62, husband, colon*

▶ Yes, once Mom yelled at me to stop helping her, but you could tell she was frustrated. *Rue, 29, mother, breast*

▶ He did seem to appreciate whatever I did for him and expressed his appreciation more than once. *Rose, 70, husband, lymphoma*

▸ No, she needed to maintain a certain degree of familiarity in attempting to live as normally as she possibly could. *Annamarie, 62, daughter, NA*

▸ Sometimes but I didn't stop trying to help. He would criticize, and I would give it right back (not hurtful)! *Lynn, 64, brother, colon*

▸ He could get really "short" if the answer wasn't what he wanted to hear, and I would get hurt feelings. *Patti, 52, husband, kidney*

▸ No, there were times when there was too much help and she needed to do things herself. *Leonard, 41, wife, breast*

▸ At first I was not aware, but after calling the Cancer Center, I was comfortable doing what I could. *Barbara, 61, aunt, breast*

▸ Never. She was very independent and I encouraged her to remain so. *N, 68, friend, breast*

▸ Probably not until the last couple of weeks before he died, and then only because of total mental and physical exhaustion. *Lisa, 40, husband, brain*

▸ No, I understand the need to feel "normal," independent. *Diane, 38, friend/co-worker, breast*

▸ As her husband, I was supposed to fix things and make things better. You can't do that if your advice is ignored or turned down. *Mark, 45, wife, breast*

▸ Sometimes, but I realized I had to let her come to me. I didn't want to be the type of friend who smothered her, or thought she couldn't do something. *Barb, 44, best friend, non-Hodgkins lymphoma*

▸ I always offered to let her live with us. She refused until her final hospital stay, then asked to come to our home. *Sharon, 65, friend, breast*

"Help was never turned down by the patient. At times her family had trouble with her calling (us). We could let her be honest with us. Her family could not." *Mary, 63, best friend, breast*

Just one of many

Giving help without pushing too much

This is a challenge at times, how well your friends and the family are willing to accept help. Initially it can be very difficult to accept assistance with things you are used to doing yourself. Some people feel a sense of pride by "doing it themselves," but often if an illness is extended, this feeling tends to fade.

Speaking as someone who has gone through this process, it is a "gift" to be able to accept love and help from others without wondering "why are they doing all this for me?" Realizing that many people just want to make things easier or better is an overwhelming thing to accept. At some point, you just need to start saying yes to help and let others do what they can. A spouse may feel even more uncomfortable if they have started to "take over" some of your duties and start to feel like they should "do it all." Trying to be supportive and keep everything running may work out for awhile, but eventually the stress will build up.

Giving choices for your friend, such as a list of people, types of help, etc., can be a great way to offer. Gently keep asking what is needed. If refused, let your friend change their mind and choose to accept an offer even if they had initially said no.

144

How to help a friend who is pushing everyone away

Some people go through a time when they become angry and may push friends away. It is easy to feel jealous of your friends who are "normal" and are not facing such a scary disease. They may need time to deal with their own fears and reject offers to get together or accept help. This can be very difficult to accept as you really may feel a need to remain close and do what you can for your friend.

It's not the size of the effort, but the caring thoughts that mean the most when it comes to helping out.

Robin

1Ø1 ways to help

Copy these pages and circle the things people can do for you.

1. Offer to dust the house
2. Baby-sit the children
3. Prepare meals
4. Mow the lawn
5. Run errands
6. Give rides to and from treatment visits or doctor's appointments
7. Take phone calls, or act as a phone secretary
8. Coordinate scheduling, (gifts, cards, meals)
9. Purchase gift certificates for videos, CDs, or audio tapes
10. Purchase phone cards for hospital long distance calls
11. Check on children and assist them if they want to talk about the cancer, their loved one, or what's going on in their life.
12. Walk the dog
13. Do a load of laundry
14. Relay messages to neighbors, family
15. Bring flowers
16. Give your loved one a journal so they can write down their thoughts
17. Make a photo album
18. Give a shawl
19. Take your loved one to a movie

#6
Give rides to and from treatment visits or doctor's appointments

20. Send inspirational or funny e-mails
21. Pick up prescriptions or medications at the drug store
22. Make little positive slogan or "affirmation cards"
23. Arrange a "healing service," "prayer chain," "special intentions," "healing masses"
24. Purchase McDonald's gift coupons for the children or buy local restaurant gift certificates for take out (pizza, dinners, lunch, etc).
25. Take up collections for a new hat, wig, or a stylish scarf
26. Bring gifts of aromatherapy candles
27. Bring lotion or body crème for massage or back rub
28. Bring books such as "Chicken Soup for the Soul" or Louise Hay books such as "You Can Heal Your Life."
29. Take children to run their errands or to get school supplies
30. Do grocery shopping for the survivor.
31. Help your loved one do shopping (drop off at the door, carry groceries into the house, or put them in refrigerator)
32. Ask the children to come over and play at your house, or take them to the zoo, the library or to a movie
33. Help wash hair with dry soap
34. Wait with the loved one before treatments
35. Bring handheld games (solitaire, Game Boy, etc.)
36. Help with a phone or e-mail tree to concerned friends about results, tests, progress, etc.
37. Hugs, hugs, hugs.
38. Take kids overnight or for dinner
39. Bring stuffed animals to hug
40. See if "special needs" of family can be accomplished by a group (paint garage, house repair, get holiday gifts for children)
41. Let spouse or friends answer the phone to maximize the energy of the patient. Suggest screening calls.
42. Bring funny pajamas as a gift
43. Offer to help organize medications in containers
44. Make chicken soup and bring a Chicken Soup book to accompany the soup

#29
Take children to run their errands or to get school supplies

45. Make a poster board of pictures with the slogan, "We love you!"
46. Help prepare for holidays (run errands, get gifts, get valentines, cards at the store, make a turkey, etc).
47. Polish nails, give a pedicure, or a massage
48. Shovel the driveway
49. Plant some flowers in the yard
50. Purchase inspirational or funny books

147

51. Bring cartoons or VCR tapes of funny television shows to laugh together
52. Visit and read a book to the survivor
53. Bring over hot chamomile tea and laugh and joke about old times
54. Do a puzzle together
55. Drive the survivor to a cancer support group
56. Help the survivor make a list of priorities or a "to-do list"
57. Help survivors catch up with mail and correspondence
58. Send cards, e-mails or post-cards

> #51
> Bring cartoons or VCR tapes of funny TV shows to laugh together

59. Visit the survivor at home or in the hospital
60. Help with tasks around the house
61. Pray
62. Bring over magazines or calming CD's
63. Bring cookies and fruit for survivor's family and visitors
64. Offer to drive your loved one to treatments or appointments
65. Send flowers
66. Offer support and encouragement
67. Offer to shave your head as an act of solidarity
68. Open your heart and just "listen" to the survivor
69. Celebrate life with your loved one
70. Use humor, jokes, or gag gifts to help your survivor laugh
71. Make a donation to a cancer-related organization in honor of your loved one
72. Invite the survivor and partner over for dinner
73. Talk to the survivor, but try not to dwell on the diagnosis

74. Give a gift certificate for a day at a spa or a free massage
75. Bring over breakfast or muffins
76. Offer to join the survivor at the annual Race for the Cure
77. Give religious medals as a gift of hope
78. Be positive
79. Offer to stay at the survivors home overnight to help with medical concerns
80. Accept the diagnosis
81. Vacuum
82. Start a hospital-wide bone marrow drive
83. Respect their need to work or stay busy
84. Take your loved one out to lunch
85. Give lots of kisses
86. Offer unconditional acceptance
87. Assist with paying bills if money is tight
88. Help the survivor with filling out insurance or Medicare claims
89. Give inspirational books
90. Help the survivor with keeping up with their accounting/bills
91. Offer to take the survivor to reflexology, yoga classes, or meditation
92. Treat your survivor normally
93. Create a healing quilt
94. Give your loved one a survivor's "cancer bear"
95. Take the survivor for a ride in your car or convertible
96. Help them with correspondence or work by setting up a computer connection for them at home
97. Cry with them
98. Make a video of friends, children, students, or other friends and family offering supportive comments
99. Send news clips of relevant information
100. Make them know they are loved
101. Take your survivor for coffee to your favorite coffee shop

#72
Invite the survivor and partner over for dinner

Top responses

- Make a phone call and check in with your loved one
- Send cards, e-mails or postcards
- Visit them at home or in the hospital
- Pray for them
- Offer support & encouragement

My friends can

- _____
- _____
- _____
- _____
- _____
- _____
- _____

50 ways friends can help

1. Be there! Cancer patients frequently talk about losing friends after they hear about their diagnosis. Reach out; silence hurts more than anything else.

2. Deliver encouragement and inspiration to your loved one. They need your positive reinforcement and uplifting behavior.

3. Be cautious of appearing judgmental of decisions on treatment choices.

4. Send cards of support to your loved one.

5. Listen. Let your loved one share their feelings without judgment. Listen with your heart, and not your head.

6. Talk about life, not just the cancer.

7. Choose words carefully. (Avoid statements such as: "I know how you feel," "Well, you did smoke" or "Didn't you see the warning signs?")

8. Offer assistance to caregivers so they can get away from responsibilities for a short period of time. Perhaps you can stay in the hospital room so a caregiver can go home and take a nap, or perhaps help at home so they can have some time for themselves.

9. Be sensitive to the loved one's coping styles. Their style for coping may not be your way, but they may work for the cancer patient.

10. Respect decisions of your loved one (chemotherapy, etc). You don't have to like the decisions, but just let them choose.

11. Promote hope. Look for opportunities, and point them out.

12. Say it directly, "I'm sorry to hear about your cancer ..."

13. Help to keep life "as it was" or as close to "normal" as much as possible.

14. Be honest with feelings, but don't overburden your loved one with your own feelings.

#13

Help to keep life "as it was" or as close to "normal" as much as possible

151

15. Give hugs. Make sure your body language is open and supportive.

16. Be a source of stability ... things may change, but no matter what, let them know you are there.

17. Try to be positive and the fun person who makes visits enjoyable (bring bubbles, coloring books, etc.)

18. Offer to do specific tasks. Remember that most people won't ask for your help.

19. Offer to research online websites, journals articles, or community resources to assist with decision making in treatment.

20. Ask if you can share information about the cancer prognosis with others. Remember your loved one has the right to the decision of whether they want their information shared with others.

21. Create an opening to discuss the cancer. Perhaps you could open the conversation with: "I don't know much about cancer, but I'm sure this has been so difficult. Would you like to talk about it?"

22. Be assertive. Try to be direct in your communication with your loved love. Try saying something such as: "I know I keep offering to help and you say no, but how about if I drop off dinner, pick up the kids for two hours, or bring you some movies?"

23. Your loved one needs to hear they are working hard to fight against the diagnosis. Remember to say things that reinforce their personal journey such as: "You look so healthy and strong."

24. Give positive reinforcement such as: "You've been an inspiration to more people than you could ever know."

25. Share your spiritual support with comments such as: "You are in my prayers."

26. Try to be calming and supportive.

27. Allow your loved one time alone with their family and time to be alone with their own thoughts.

28. Don't deny the reality of the diagnosis. Allow the loved one time to share their "real" feelings, even if those feelings are difficult to hear.

29. Help your loved one set small goals to create success. Reassure them by saying, "You can do it ..."

30. Learn about the stages of grief. Be aware there are times when the patient will be angry, depressed, bargaining, and accepting of the disease. Just *be there* and listen and realize the feelings are not directed at you.

31. Be there, even if it hurts.

32. Talk to a support person or counselor if you need to work through your own feelings. Don't stuff your own feelings and create disharmony within yourself.

33. Remember that many loved ones feel "different" and isolated from daily life. Cancer patients repeatedly state they want to be treated like the same person they were before the diagnosis.

34. Help create a support team of professionals who can assist with knowledge.

35. Do some research, perhaps through pamphlets or online to know a little about the disease. Knowledge helps your conversation and understanding when talking to your loved one.

#34
Help create a support team of professionals who can assist with knowledge

36. You could help them by screening their phone calls, relaying information or assigning a friend to relay information to concerned friends and family.

37. Call to say "I'm just thinking of you" and if you receive an answering machine message add, "There is no need to call back, I just wanted you to know you are on my mind today."

38. If you have had difficulty calling a loved one, you might call and say something like: "I'm sorry it took so long for me to call, but I have to tell you I just didn't know what to say except that I care about (love) you."

153

39. Place an updated message on the answering machine to give new information on the status of the loved one. Perhaps you can say something like: "We will return calls as energy permits. We appreciate your call and it means so much to us."

40. If you write a card put in something positive like: "I'm looking forward to spending some time with you." Talk about resiliency, their strength or courage.

41. Say things to the loved one such as: "I love you," "It's okay to cry," "You don't have to be cheerful with me, you can let down and talk about your feelings," or "Don't worry, I'm here for you no matter what."

42. Take your loved one to a restorative yoga class or suggest going to a meditation class to help them find "peaceful time" with themselves.

43. Ask your loved one if they would like you to read to them, or draw cartoons.

44. Bring board games or cards to help the survivor through difficult days in the hospital, during chemotherapy, or at home.

45. Make sure you remember to touch the survivor. Many survivors feel isolated, alien, untouchable, "damaged" or afraid.

#42
Take your loved one to a restorative yoga class or suggest going to a meditation class to help them find peaceful time with themselves

46. Sit with the survivor's family in the waiting room of hospitals or treatment offices. Remember that cancer affects the whole family.

47. Be cautious of chemicals, perfumes, or other toxins that may create discomfort or reactions for the survivor.

48. Create a ball cap or scarf wrap with your survivor. Wear an identical one in solidarity.

49. Drive the survivor to the Race for the Cure, the American Cancer Society's Relay for Life or other cancer events, and walk with them. Afterward, go out and celebrate their survivorship, resiliency, and perseverance.

50. Listen with your heart, speak through your soul, and touch the person who needs you!

Ways to help me

✎ _____

✎ _____

✎ _____

✎ _____

✎ _____

✎ _____

✎ _____

✎ _____

✎ _____

Flowers: They'll love them, they'll love them not

Should I send flowers or not? That's one of the great mysteries of life when you want to send get well greetings. Some people love them at times like this, but a flood of flowers reminds others of a funeral home.

When sending or delivering flowers or plants, keep in mind what kind of care they'll need. If they require a lot of attention, that may put too many demands on the patient/survivor and their family.

Keep in mind any allergies or medical restrictions. You also have to consider the fragrance. The patient may be more sensitive to certain scents, and that may deter from their beauty. Below are some low-fragrance, yet still beautiful plants as gifts:

Azalea, hydrangea, shamrocks, tulips, pansies, lisianthus, daisies, African violet, alstroemeria (Princess Lily), sunflower, anthurium (Hawaiian Love Plant), cyclamen, cineraria, bird-of-paradise, kalanchoe, exacum (Persian violet), calla, some orchids, primrose, gerbera, anemone, ginger, banksias, Belles of Ireland, amaryllis, dahlia and *begonia.*

Some foliage plants have great color and texture, but no fragrance include *peperomia, arrowhead, coleus* and *spider plant.*

Extremely fragrant plants/flowers that you might want to avoid include *lilies,* some *orchids, gladiolus,* and unfortunately, the ever-popular *roses* and *carnations.*

> "Send cards. Don't send flowers. My home looked and smelled like a funeral home. Not good."
> Kathy, 61, breast

> "Send cards and flowers. I love flowers." Maria, 61, breast

155

Just one of many

156

▸ "I really appreciated it when people would ask first before they told other people. I felt like they were really respecting our feelings by doing this."

▸ "I got so many calls initially that I changed my answering machine message to say 'thanks for calling, I will call you back when time and energy permits.' I wanted to know that people cared about me, but it was just too much to be constantly on the phone."

▸ "I always thought it was so hard to share my bad news with others. Once someone knew, it made it much easier to talk about the situation. I had one really close friend who I would talk to first, then she would start a calling chain to others. This worked well so that no one had to repeat the details too often, yet people who really wanted to know could keep up on things."

▸ "We know almost all friends mean well and would never do things to hurt their friends, especially at this time. However, sometimes it just doesn't turn out quite right!"

Robin & friends

If they say stay away, it's nothing personal!

We know you want to help the survivor. However, there is a fine line between assistance and invasion. What do we mean by that? This is a hard one to define, but somewhere in the middle there is a place where you can visit a loved one, and then it becomes too much and it feels uncomfortable for the survivor and the family. One of our care-givers told us, "It's a fine line, but sometimes it feels like people kept invading our home. Sometimes, we just needed some time for us."

As we said, this can be a difficult balance to define because a primary caretaker may not want visitors, while the survivor wants loved ones surrounding them. Children may need to maintain a constant routine with eating, homework, and other nighttime events, but loved ones want to come and see the cancer survivor. What if the survivor is fatigued and wants to spend time alone, but is too timid to hurt people's feelings by saying "Please don't come over tonight"? What if the survivor and their significant other just want one night alone to themselves?

Here are some suggestions to assist with the "fine line":

▸ *Consider making a time period where you'd prefer not to have visitors.* Perhaps one night a week? Quiet time after 8:30 or 9 p.m.?

▸ *Be direct with loved ones if you are fatigued, or don't want visitors.* Your loved ones will appreciate your honesty

▸ *Try to maintain a normal schedule for children.* They need con-sistent times to study, have alone time with their parent, and time to relax. You can always have one parent spend time with the children, while the other one talks to visitors.

▸ *Be honest and introspective about your priorities.* If you don't want visitors on a certain night, you can put a message on your answering machine saying "We're spending time alone tonight, hope to talk to you tomorrow."

▸ *Be honest with your significant other and discuss the issues of inclusion versus invasion.* Together create a plan that works for both of your needs.

▸ *Create a "do not disturb" sign that can be placed on your front door during down times.*

We know you want to help, but... HELP!

Robin Unes' original title for the book she wanted to write was a simple, yet effective "Laughter & Lasagna." Laughter you need lots of, lasagna you don't.

Robin's family wasn't the first or last family to be inundated by the generosity of loved ones and friends when it comes to food. Survivors and family have told us of being overwhelmed by trays, buckets and baskets of homemade goodies. They're much appreciated, but not just all at once or the only dish you know how to prepare with great love and expertise.

In the preparation of all the ingredients for this book, we discovered a new definition of the word casserole: *Something people quickly get sick of.*

For those of you who want to help a family dealing with cancer or other serious illness by providing meals, consider the following suggestions:

▶ *Put one person in charge of meals by using a schedule on the facing page to coordinate who will be bringing what when.* This will avoid duplication of food and make sure all days are filled according to the family's needs.

▶ *Remember that the usual home refrigerator and freezer will only hold so much.* Consider making smaller portions instead of enough to feed an army. That's easier on the family because they won't have to worry about storing leftovers.

▶ *Ask the family what they really want to eat and what they never want to see again.* Yes, your dish may be the best of its kind in the world, but they're going to tire of it pretty soon.

▶ *If you really want or need to cook up a storm to cope with cancer, call a local social agency that provides food for needy people in your community.* Perhaps you can prepare a big meal in honor of the cancer survivor.

And don't forget the ever-popular gift certificate to the family's favorite take-out restaurant, preferably one that delivers!

Cancer: Here's how YOU can help ME cope & survive

Meal schedule

159

Day	Who's bringing	What	Phone number
Sun __/__			
Mon __/__			
Tues __/__			
Wed __/__			
Thurs __/__			
Fri __/__			
Sat __/__			
Sun __/__			
Mon __/__			
Tues __/__			
Wed __/__			
Thurs __/__			
Fri __/__			
Sat __/__			

It's okay to say 'NO!'

160

"There is a fine line between being cordial and being rude. All the people are coming over and sometimes I wanted to say, 'NO, don't bring us dinner.' I had a mat at the door that said, 'Go away!' Everyone felt like they wanted to do something. It was a normal reaction. Everybody's involved in so many groups. All of us have a need to help because it's human nature. But be careful about how often people come over. The primary caregiver has to draw the line. Learn to say 'NO,' though it's rough to get to that point. Saying 'NO' is not to hurt people. We just need some time for us."

L, wife, breast

Simple additions and ideas can make food more appealing

161

"I'm not hungry … nothing tastes good."

Loved ones are likely going to hear that a lot from the cancer survivor as they undergo treatment. Medications, radiation and chemotherapy can play havoc with the body while attempting to eradicate the disease. Caregivers and friends must remember that their role is providing the food but accepting the fact that they can't force the survivor to eat.

One survivor explains that "It's like being pregnant. You don't know what you want, and you don't like what you get."

Though you should follow your doctor's orders, you might want to keep the following dietary notes in mind:

▶ *The appetite will generally decrease during treatments.* Small amounts of food at shorter intervals will be tolerated better than three larger meals a day.

▶ *Tart flavors, such as fruit or juices and even sucking on pickles, can stimulate the taste buds and appetite.*

▶ *Fruits and juices can be added to other foods to make them taste better, i.e. sauces.*

▶ *Fruit juices should be avoided in case of mouth sores.* Consider bland foods such as mashed potatoes, pureed foods, cream soups, cottage cheese, pudding, custard and eggs. These offer protein and are easy to consume when you can't chew.

"Don't cook anything you wouldn't want to smell if you had morning sickness. Ha ha ha." Gresha, 47, breast

▶ *Avoid salty foods and straws while dealing with mouth sores.*

▶ *To get more calories into limited amounts of food, add margarine or cheese, which can also add flavor.* Consider other condiments like salsa, cottage cheese, yogurt or peanut butter.

▶ *Add more flavor and calories to basic foods with fruit dips or peanut butter.*

162

▶ *Ginger ale can help clear the taste buds.*

▶ *If certain unpleasant tastes linger, try sucking on a lemon or mint or chew gum.*

▶ *If the survivor has developed an aversion to meat or poultry, marinade it first.* Try it in fruit juice, wine or a vinegar-based salad dressing to enhance the flavor.

"My son baked me cinnamon raisin bread when food sounded terrible."
Elaine, 72, leukemia

▶ *Lemon or strawberry Italian ice can be satisfying if the survivor has no appetite.*

▶ *Milk products, such as cheese, yogurt and yogurt drinks, are an excellent source of protein.* This is essential to repairing damaged tissues. A milk shake can often be tolerated.

▶ *Add a drink powder to give something bland a little more flavor.*

Stimulating a cancer survivor's appetite is more than just the type of food. It's also a matter or timing, portions and setting.

▶ *Instead of regular meals, try stimulating a survivor's appetite with "eating by the clock."* It's okay even if they consume only one type of food at one time. If you wait for the survivor to be hungry, you may be waiting an awfully long time.

▶ *Don't set a full plate of food in front of the survivor.* It can be overwhelming. Try smaller quantities in smaller bowls or plates

▶ *Serve the survivor with plastic utensils.* Certain treatments may leave a nasty metallic taste in their mouths, and regular silverware can worsen that sensation.

▶ *Make one-dish meals, such as a cream soup with meat added.*

▶ *Change the surroundings.* Maybe the survivor doesn't want to eat at the table where loved ones will be "monitoring" how much they consume. Dining in the front of the television may offer a diversion from the pressure to eat.

▸ *A survivor may rebel against eating if caregivers pressure them.* Coax but don't force. Give them lots of choices. If they refuse, just be politely persistent and supportive, because their bodies are being stressed both emotionally and physically in extremes most of can't even imagine.

163

▸ *If certain smells bother the survivor, consider serving foods at room temperature or cold because that reduces the aroma.* Using a slow cooker fills the house with fewer smells than traditional cooking methods.

▸ *If the weather's nice, go outside to eat if the survivor wants to.*

▸ *If the survivor becomes nauseated, let them try eating solid foods without liquid, or serve beverages between meals to keep the stomach from churning.*

▸ *Covering a cup of liquid and drinking through a straw can cut down on the smell.*

What sounds good?

- _____
- _____
- _____
- _____
- _____
- _____
- _____

Friends need to understand, be honest and willing to listen

Kathy Burdon learned the hard way when to push, when to be a "pain in the ass" and when to be honest when her dear friend, Diane Cullinan Oberhelman, battled an aggressive form of breast cancer in 1995.

She knows what it's like to lose a loved one to cancer. A sister lost the fight, and her mother also had cancer. Those experiences prepared her for the emotional support Diane wanted and needed.

When diagnosed, Diane hesitated asking her friends for assistance. Kathy found out from someone else about her cancer and contacted her. The reality of the treatment and her disease had started to take its toll on the patient.

Kathy joined her the day after her mastectomy and visited again several times before Diane went to Iowa City for the stem cell transplant in October 1995. She saw her after the chemotherapy and remembers sitting on the bed while Diane apologized for feeling so lousy.

"I would just hang out and find out if there was anything I could do. She was definitely into the foot rub." Kathy laughs.

However, the patient felt guilty. "Kathy had a job. She couldn't drop everything," Diane says. "I went through a period where I was really discouraged, which is unusual for me."

Kathy took Diane's parents' place in caring for their daughter for short periods in Iowa City, Iowa. "The most difficult part was watching how this was affecting everyone else. Knowing I could talk to Kathy and she would not be judgmental ... it was really helpful to take care of things if something would happen. I finally came to the realization that I was a lot sicker than I thought."

Kathy nods.

Lesson #1
Survivors want you around, but not too much

"They want you to be honest, but they don't want to feel like aliens either. They want you around, but not too much," Kathy explains. Diane would say things like, "I don't want to ruin your day," but being responsive and speaking up helped both of them. The cancer patient needs someone to be there for anything.

Kathy doesn't regret a moment of the time she spent with her.

"I was glad I was there in Iowa. I knew what the procedure was and how nasty it could be. Sometimes you just have to go." When she first saw her, "I thought she looked okay. She was just trying to be Diane. She woke up and smiled, and we all laughed and took pictures of ourselves in the garb." They talked about a wide range of topics, including how cancer had quickly taught Diane how to focus on the true priorities in her life, family and friends, after such a hectic pre-cancer life. "That was a shift I saw in her that came out of all of this.

"You just have to be there and listen," Kathy says. "Sometimes they lead you a little and give you an opening. Sometimes they shut the door on you. But you can't take it personally. That's probably the hardest part." What they loved 10 minutes earlier, like a foot rub, may bother them later. You just have to remember that and "not let it get into your spirit. Just keep coming back." The fax machine was a lifesaver as she could keep in touch with jokes and other words of support when she couldn't be there.

Lesson #2
Sometimes survivors lead you a little and give you an opening

165

One weekend, the same tape ran seven times. Kathy explains that the rhythm of the movie helped Diane relax and fall asleep. They laugh now at that endless weekend.

Yet, another critical time came when Diane faced a fungal infection without an immune system to protect her. Kathy calls that her personal low point. "That really scared me, and I wasn't there. This was very touch-and-go treatment."

During that marathon movie weekend, Kathy describes Diane as lucid before her condition worsened. "She was somebody who needed to talk. She wanted things to be affirmed."

Diane nods. "I was genuinely scared. It hit me that something could happen. I desperately needed to know that someone was hearing me." She wanted to make sure that someone else, in addition to their father, was an advocate for her four children and knew her wishes, such as fulfilling their college choices and other aspects of their future. "I thought Kathy was the one to fill the role. It gave me comfort knowing that someone knew how I thought and felt."

Kathy says some people think the conversation is an admission that death is going to happen. However, you don't have to be morbid to talk about important issues. It's too often a taboo subject.

Diane believes in the theory that it's not a matter of whether there is adversity in life, but when and how you handle it. Kathy would just be another person there when her children reached those forks in the road, to answer the kids when they'd ask, "What would Mom think?"

Kathy remembers the positive Diane during that period.

"She tried to keep her life and their lives as normal as possible. Maybe that wasn't completely right, but a large part of that worked well." It added to her peace of mind. "There was that constant drive, 'We're going to keep going forward.' " She didn't want the world to stop because she had cancer, Kathy adds. "That was the thing she loved most, all of them hanging out together watching a movie at home," while recovering from her transplant.

"She had to go through her own process … If you can't read a cancer patient, just say, 'I can't really tell how you're feeling right now, but I'd like to do this for you. Would that bother you?'

"For Diane, it was a curse and a gift, and she was able to learn something from the cancer and absorb it in a positive way. That was amazing to see and be part of," particularly how she's touched other people's lives in sharing her battle with cancer.

Lesson #3
You don't have to be morbid to talk about important issues

Please write me! One liners for get well cards

Don't know what to do when someone you care about is diagnosed with cancer? A simple card can mean volumes to the patient. Don't know what to say? There are lots of ready-made cards, but here are short snippets to help you write your own.

- Best wishes for a full and speedy recovery
- You are in our prayers
- Sending along a hug and my love
- I know you will never give up
- I know you are a survivor
- Wishing you much peace and comfort
- Happy healing!
- Remember you are not alone, and you are loved by so many
- You are in our thoughts
- You are a fighter and I know cancer will not win
- I'm concerned about you, and wanted you to know how much you mean to me
- I'm hoping you are feeling better after your treatments
- I am inspired by the way you are handling your diagnosis
- You are an inspiration to me
- I admire your strength and resiliency
- I just heard about the diagnosis and wanted you to know I cared
- The office is not the same without you … hurry back!
- You were in my thoughts today, and I just wanted to drop you a note and tell you "I love you"
- You have been on my mind and in my heart
- Work is not the same without you, but we are pulling together and doing some extra things anticipating your return
- Things will soon become manageable. Just take one step at a time. I will walk with you through it all.

Don't smother me!

168

"If someone is not up to visitors, or going out somewhere, respect their wishes; it doesn't necessarily mean we're down or depressed."
Lorraine, 48, breast

"If the cancer patient doesn't feel like having company, don't take it person- ally. They may just be having a bad day."
Tracy, 47, mother, lung

"Do not smother. Keep up natural relations. Be real. B consistent, not pile on, then pull away o opposite." V, 66, breast

"Just be there for them for anything they need, but don't invade their space."
Clint, 48, wife, breast

Creating stronger relationships

"Tell them to talk when they are hurting or scared." Melinda, 46, breast

Ways parents can assist adult children

Some of our strongest responses came from parents whose children developed cancer. For most parents, the thought of a child developing a potentially life-threatening disease is a crisis of a monumental magnitude. As parents, many believed they would be the one who would need a caregiver, and not the other way around.

Whether the child was in their twenties, thirties, forties or older, our survey indicated an affiliation and bonding between child and parent that goes beyond words. Faced with the crisis, our parents spoke of their powerful connection to their children, and their effort to assist them in their battle with cancer. With love, compassion, and tenderness, you will view some of the ways in which our parents assisted their children.

Here are their suggestions of how to help your child:

▶ Be positive about the diagnosis, treatment options, and the future

▶ Be supportive and encouraging

▶ Offer a "take charge" attitude to assist with tasks

▶ Make daily phone calls to check in with the survivor

▶ Pray for your loved one

▶ Openly cry with your child, illustrating the importance of being open with emotions

▶ Make frequent visits to the survivor

▶ Bring little gifts to the survivor

▶ Encourage normality by acting as if the future would be okay

▶ Drive them to treatments, physician appointments and the hospital

▶ Stay with them at their house to give medical care and support

▶ Tell them about their innerstrength and power to "beat" cancer

▶ Help with meals for the significant other and grandchildren

▶ Listen, listen, listen

▶ Give hugs

▶ Help them laugh

- Bring over inspirational tapes and books
- Remind them of the way they coped in the past
- Talk about ways they achieved success in the past
- Take care of grandchildren
- Be a positive role model
- Encourage them to get out and participate in activities
- E-mail daily devotions and words of encouragement each day
- Tell them " I love you"

- Assist by making meals
- Pick up medications at the pharmacy
- Run errands
- Assist financially with treatments
- Taking time away from work to assist
- Assist with household tasks
- Do some laundry
- Help the grandchildren with homework

|7|

'We knew she would never give up'

Diane Oberhelman's parents, Fred and Tilley Allen, recall the "devastating experience of having Diane, who we love beyond words, unexpectedly stricken with cancer. We knew that she would think, 'Why would this happen?' and we felt the same. We also knew that Diane would never give up. She had so much to live for and didn't want to leave her three daughters, son and family …

"As parents with heavy and grieving hearts, we knew we would do everything in our power to support our precious daughter and her family. We understood the course of treatment. One of us would be at her side every minute of the day and night. She suffered so … We applied ice packs all night and throughout the day (to control fevers). We were so afraid, but tried to stay strong. It's so very important for the patient. Being there, praying and hoping the strength from your love and very being would help. We still feel the hurt of her illness as it penetrated us … Her severe pain and sickness was overwhelming. She would smile and say, 'I'm so sorry,' as though she was causing problems for others. She'd say, 'I'm trying so hard.'

"I'd try to have the children be quieter sometimes. She didn't want them quiet. She wanted them to be themselves, yell and laugh. … If someone you love is very ill, the thing that is most important is giving your time, love, care. Never feel rushed. Try to give them strength and encourage them to push and accomplish what the doctor ordered. We are so grateful for her wonderful health."

To my child

Dear

Watching you endure this terrible disease absolutely breaks my heart. No matter how old you are, you're still my child, and I will never stop loving and caring for you.

I know you're scared, even when you put on that brave face I know so well. And I'm scared, too. Sometimes I am so frustrated that I can't do more for you because I would do anything for you. But I know that sometimes all you need is for me to just sit beside you, listen or hold your hand. I hope that by being with you that I can give you some kind of strength and sense of security.

You'll always have my love and my heart, and my promise to be there for you, to help you during this difficult battle.

Love,

Survivors say...

What did your parents do or say to assist you?

▶ My mom is a survivor, so I had her as an example of what I was in for. She was very helpful with her knowledge. *Robin, 46, breast*

▶ My mom prayed and cried. *Kathy, 61, breast*

▶ Unfortunately both of my parents died of cancer, my father at age 52 from liver/colon cancer, and my mom at age 72 from lung cancer. *Jim, 50, thyroid*

▶ They were always there, and they stayed strong and it made me stay strong. They had a take-charge and fighting attitude, and it made me move that way. *Mary Ann, 56, colon*

▶ Even though they lived out of town, they would come whenever I had to go to the hospital. Phone calls to check on me and my mom's great humor. *Mary, 52, breast*

▶ My dad was suffering from the loss of my mother and from prostate cancer as well. He did like to visit and talk. *Rita, 58, breast*

▶ My mother worried a lot and wished it was her instead of me. I didn't want her to know too much. *Bill, 64, throat and tongue*

▶ Nothing. *Paula, 53, uterine and breast*

▶ Brought me little gifts to surprise me. *Sandy, 58, breast*

▶ My 98-year-old mother was still living when I had treatments. She carried on in a nursing home until I was better. Then she died after I was better. *Helen, 71, lymphoma*

▶ Lived as if I would be fine. *Karen, 33, breast*

▶ Mother deceased from lung cancer in 1997. Father was by my side every step of the way. *Diana, 46, lung*

▶ Took care of the children, called often. *S, 61, breast*

▶ Mom visited me even though it was hard for her to leave Dad one afternoon with a home helper. *Martha, 51, breast*

- My mother had Alzheimer's, so she never really understood. My dad was there for me, very supportive and a good listener. *Julie, 61, breast*

- They reminded me to stay in touch with my usual, positive attitude and fighting nature. They believed I could survive. *Jennifer, 42, breast*

174

- Well, not much. They are old school. They think "cancer" and the world should stop spinning because you're close to the six-foot under mark. Hopefully I've showed them not to give up. *Sara, 35, lung*

- They had a hard time dealing with the whole thing. My mother had a heart attack. *Carol, 71, colon*

- My mother quit her job for three and a half months to take care of me and my daughters. *Ana, 35, breast*

- My parents were sad for me at first, and my mom always wished it would have been her instead of me. Four years down the road, she discovered she had it, too. *Vicki, 53, breast*

- My father was dying of bone cancer. We hugged, talked and cried and prayed together. *JoAnn, breast*

- My parents "looked after me." I felt protected by them. My mother was with me for all my chemotherapy treatments, and my father is a retired surgeon, so he rallied the medical troops. *Ann, 45, breast*

- Being the baby of five, my parents felt my pain. They were always there with their unconditional love (and food). Also, they were hungry for more information on eternal life, so it was great to share what I understood. *Cheryl, 48, rectal*

- My dad was always there whenever I was in the hospital. I would wake up in the morning, and he would be at the foot of my bed. *Lori, 39, melanoma*

"My father, with whom I lived, criticized my sleeping long periods of time and complained about my hair on the bathroom floor when it was falling out."
J, 25, lymphoma

Ways children can assist their parents 175

Adult children

Many people have been faced with their parent being diagnosed with cancer. The roles now may be reversed, and many children feel like they now become the caregivers to those who cared for them. But, children have the opportunity to "give back" in many ways to their parent who cared for them whether emotionally, spiritually, or physically.

Here are some suggestions for adult children of survivors and young children whose parents have cancer:

- Just "be there" for support and encouragement
- Provide love
- Drive survivor to appointments and treatments
- Help around the house with tasks
- Provide lots of hugs
- Help to keep the survivor active
- Provide emotional support
- Maintain a positive attitude
- Provide a goal or purpose for living (to see grandchildren, be at a wedding, make it to a specific event, etc.)
- Call on the telephone to say hello
- Make dinners or lunches
- Be attentive to needs
- Advocate for them with the physician or heath care workers
- Send cards of encouragement and love
- Bring pets to the house to provide love
- Pray for and with the survivor
- Help with dressings due to medical issues
- Help with bathing
- Help with needs that are important to the survivor
- Stay overnight to assist with needs
- Help gather information on cancer, treatment options, physicians, etc.

176

- ▶ Take them to your house for care
- ▶ Encourage them to "never give up"
- ▶ Help select wigs and hats
- ▶ Insure that life is as "normal" as possible
- ▶ Make the survivor laugh
- ▶ Clean the house
- ▶ Just sit and be with them
- ▶ Give "tender loving care"
- ▶ Attend a caregiver support group
- ▶ Keep the lines of communication open
- ▶ Talk to them about their wishes concerning treatment
- ▶ Be open to listen to them about their wishes concerning wills, estates, living wills, etc.
- ▶ Help them create a priority list of what they would like accomplished

- ▶ Help them respond to cards or phone calls
- ▶ Create medication boxes to assist with daily prescriptions
- ▶ Assist with insurance bills or catching up on other bills
- ▶ Send them e-mails
- ▶ Say "I love you"
- ▶ Let them know you will be there for them
- ▶ Make chicken soup
- ▶ Take them out for dinner
- ▶ Stay with them so the other parent can get out for a while by themselves
- ▶ Bring over picture of the kids
- ▶ Bring the children over to visit and spend some time with their grandparent(s)
- ▶ Take the dog or cat to the vet or run errands

Top responses

- ✎ Just 'be there'
- ✎ Phone to say hi & check in
- ✎ Provide love and encouragement
- ✎ Be a healthcare advocate
- ✎ Maintain positive attitude

Young children and teens can...

- Just "be there" for support and encouragement
- Provide love
- Help around the house with tasks
- Provide lots of hugs
- Draw pictures
- Make cards
- Make a bouquet by collecting flowers from the yard
- Make dinners or lunches
- Pray for and with the survivor
- Design a ball cap, hat, or scarf for them to wear
- Make them laugh
- Clean the house
- Just sit and be with them
- Give "tender loving care"
- Get involved with groups such as Kids Konnected (for young children and teens)
- Make a snack or dessert
- Go with them to the movie
- Take them outside and sit in the sun
- Just sit and tell stories
- Make them a photo album
- Make tea or hot chocolate
- Tuck them in bed
- Do puzzles together
- Send them e-mails
- Send them pictures or text messages from your cell phone for encouragement
- Say "I love you"
- Read to them
- Ask them to tell about funny things that happened in their life
- Share things that happened during the day
- Snuggle in bed together
- Try to stay quiet in the house when the parent is resting
- Keep up your grades
- Help with taking care of younger siblings
- Try not to get into trouble
- Get along better with siblings
- Take out the garbage
- Talk about the future
- Help write thank you notes
- Do computer searches for needed information
- Give kisses
- Run errands (groceries, drug store, etc.)
- Keep them updated on what's going on at school
- Treat them "normally"
- Drive them to get an ice cream cone

177

Open dialogue brings family closer

Lorraine's sons, then ages 19 and 18, helped in many ways, including giving her rides and picking up prescriptions. They kept an open dialogue after her diagnosis as she and her husband explained everything and told them to not be afraid to ask anything. One was in his senior year of high school, and Lorraine didn't want his only memories of that time to be of her illness. Being able to focus on her children helped her at the same time, something that gave her more energy to beat cancer.

Honesty empowers the kids

Now an adult, Maureen Cullinan looks back on the time when her mom was battling cancer, "Kids know when they are not getting the full story. It makes them feel powerless. I think giving them the truth (whether it be harsh at times or not) can empower kids to communicate more, express more emotion, and really learn from a situation. I imagine if my mom had died during her stem cell transplant, I think I would have had a lot of frustration that she did not disclose everything and that I did not react appropriately because I was off in la-la land thinking she was at a spa."

Hey kids!

✐ _____

✐ _____

✐ _____

✐ _____

✐ _____

✐ _____

✐ _____

To my parent

Dear

After all you've done for me and given me all my life, it's so hard to witness your battle against this terrible disease. But no matter what, I'm here to help you in any way I can.

It's OK to admit you're scared. Even though you're my parent, you're still a human being who feels pain and needs help. Your strength continues to inspire me as I learn more about you every day.

You must not be afraid to ask for my assistance. It doesn't mean you're weak. And you don't always have to put on a brave face for me. I'll understand.

I know that sometimes all you need is for me to just sit beside you, listen or hold your hand. You'll always have my love and my heart, and my promise to be there for you, to help you during this difficult battle.

Love,

Survivors say...

What did your children do or say to assist you?

▶ My daughter would go with me to chemotherapy and doctors' appointments. My son, 17, was in complete denial of the situation. *Mary, 52, breast*

▶ Drove me when I couldn't drive. Gave me a purpose to live. Made me feel loved. Encouraged me. *Theresa, 49, breast*

▶ Positive quietness. Telling me how the grandchildren will always remember me. *Bill, 64, throat and tongue*

▶ My children were at a time in their lives that they were looking to their future. *Gresha, 47, breast*

▶ Not much. Just called. I asked for no visitors. I just didn't want them to see me. *Maria, 61, breast*

▶ Called every day, "How are you doing? We love you. We need you." *Alveretta, 85, ovarian*

▶ Not much. My daughter wanted to be strong for me. She only made it worse for both of us. *Donna, 72, colon*

▶ They were too young to fully realize the truth of my illness. They were loving and concerned. *Judith, 70, breast*

▶ My daughter-in-law had just lost her mother to breast cancer and was filled with fear when I was diagnosed. *Sandy, 58, breast*

▶ Very little. When I asked for help, they did so reluctantly, too busy always. Oh, yeah, they did bring in three meals after surgery. *C, 79, breast*

▶ Researched cancer information. *Jude, 64, breast*

▶ They came to me and assisted in every way that they could. More importantly, they loved me. *Robert, 70, lung*

▶ Came to see me and helped me with getting up and walking (made me a lot). *Karen, 51, lung*

▶ Hugs, drew pictures. *S, 61, breast*

- Our adult daughter was very supportive. Once brought her new cat so we could get acquainted. *Helen, 71, lymphoma*

- Just being there and needing me to take care of them. They were 2 and newborn at the time. *Karen, 33, breast*

- She knew I have faith and determination in myself and don't depend on others. *N, 80, breast*

- They helped my husband take care of me. *Maxine, 84, lung*

8

- She was a great cheerleader. *Kathy, 61, breast*

- Our children were stunned. They were more considerate and attentive. *Jim, 50, thyroid*

- Loyalty and encouragement. *G, 81, uterine*

- Talked about future family gatherings. *T, 69, skin*

- My daughter was open and visited often. My son was here with hugs, but not as vocal as my daughter. *Robin, 46, breast*

- Recorded grandchildren's piano playing. *Helen, 72, lung*

- They would write to me, and my 3-year-old and 1-year-old grandchildren drew pictures. *Carolyn, 70, colon*

- Some traveled great distances to be with me. One went home and turned around and came back. *Carol, 71, colon*

- At the time, I had no children of my own, but my significant other did. This wonderful child helped me to live in the right here and right now. *Jennifer, 42, breast*

- Their smiles, laughter, tears and never-ending love. Their strength is so strong, I can't help but to feed off them! *Sara, 35, lung*

- My children walked through my illness with me. My daughter was 12 at the time and I thought she might be embarrassed to be with me in my wig, just the opposite hap-

"My children were scared but really wanted to help. My son, who was 17 at the time, just wanted to be with me. My youngest, who was 6, needed some reassurance, but he was good at praying!" *Ann, 45, breast*

pened. She told me how nice I looked and always wanted me to attend her events. *Noreen, 49, breast*

▸ If I wasn't pregnant, I'm sure my mom wouldn't have survived the treatment. My 13-year-old son and his grandmother have a bond that she doesn't have with her other grandchildren. *Carlene, 51, mother, breast*

▸ Draw pictures of me without hair. My girls did whatever they could to help me. *Ana, 35, breast*

▸ My son shared his concern, but one night it really hit him, and he sobbed, crying about my hair loss and worried I would die. I comforted him, but my positive words to him also helped me. *D, 42, breast*

▸ My only child was in kindergarten then first grade at the time. If I was feeling low and not liking the fact that I had a permanent colostomy, he'd say, "Get over it, Mom" and he was so right. He also patted my head and would just get me a drink without asking. *Cheryl, 48, rectal*

Talking & listening

We asked some of the children in the Kids Konnected support group at the Cancer Center for Healthy Living in Peoria about the ways in which they have coped with cancer in their family. They found relief through talking with others, reading and writing, and listening to music.

▸ I did the dishes and helped them get things around the house. Dad can't play catch like he used to. *Daniel, 10, father, pancreatic*

▸ I spent a lot of time watching my sisters. Most of the time Mom and Dad spent a lot of the time together. It makes me really upset to think that my dad is dying, and I don't let my friends come over. Kids Konnected has helped me to cope with the stress of a dying parent and how to help others in the same boat. *Rachael, 18, father, prostate*

▸ I do dishes. I lift heavy stuff for them ... It has canceled occasions we have planned. Kids Konnected has helped me deal with the cancer. *Jacob, 12, father, pancreatic*

Communication important to keeping kids informed

Looking back is not always easy, especially for four children to reflect on a time when they could have lost their mother to breast cancer. For this book, the now-adult children of Diane Cullinan Oberhelman revisited that period to examine what helped them and their family cope with the struggle.

Though the four Cullinan siblings were close, there was a natural age division between the two oldest and two youngest and how they responded. Kathleen and Maureen were 15 and 14 years old respectively in 1995 when their mom was diagnosed with breast cancer, while Alison and Allen were 11 and 9.

Kathleen remembers the news being presented in a "no big deal" tone. Their mother was quite convincing there was nothing to worry about, and it was easier to believe that version than the reality of the situation. Their grandmother, Diane's mother, Tilley Allen, later told the children during Diane's treatment, "Don't you realize how serious this is?"

They were concerned, but their mother emphasized normalcy. They went on with their daily life with their dad, school and activities, and their mom attended a local baseball game after her mastectomy as if nothing had happened.

"It was nice at first as we got used to the situation and the idea of her having cancer," Maureen explains. "I think we didn't ask that many questions because we didn't want to know the answers at first. It's not that easy to say to your mom that you know it's much more serious than she is telling you. First of all, you don't want to deflate her positive attitude. Secondly, you really just don't know. No one was telling us the really 'hard' stuff. We were very protected and sheltered."

Maureen says she didn't even talk to her friends about it because most kids don't want to be set apart by something as negative as a parent with cancer.

Kathleen concurs that there was a lot of denial as their mother tried to protect her kids, though they didn't know how much was being hidden. Though it was a morale booster for Diane, Kathleen admits now that she found no humor when friends helped Diane shave her head as her hair was falling out. Kathleen was angry and offended at the shaving festivities and felt uncomfortable but remained silent.

"I was angry more because it was even more of this 'no big deal' or 'fun' attitude. By that point, it was obvious that things were serious, and I didn't appreciate more casualness. I did force a smile occasionally because this was some sort of an outlet for her."

Maureen adds that "I think my mom and her adult friends were aware of the seriousness of the situation, but their coping mechanism was to have fun with it. As kids, I don't think we were mature enough to use humor. Or maybe we were so just so scared of all this unknown in our lives that we did not want to make jokes about it."

Diane made it sound like she was going to a spa when plans were announced for her stem cell transplant. "I wanted to believe her," Maureen says of her feelings before she learned more about what has happening. "I was once proud of my mom for being so brave and protective of me, but I was also a little hurt that she couldn't tell me the truth. Kids are aware when truths are being hidden from them, and I think it has a negative effect on them. That negative effect in my case was making me feel like a small child who could not contribute anything to the situation. I was basically being told that I could not handle the truth. "

Lesson #1
Spending time together is easy. Communication about difficult subjects is hard and needs to be forced sometime

Before she left, everyone decorated the house for Halloween, one of Diane's favorite holidays, as she wanted to be Mr. Clean, with her bald head. Maureen found the overabundance of decorations embarrassing and preferred to be dropped off at the end of the driveway so her friends wouldn't see it.

Kathleen remembers the weekly Sunday visits to their mom in isolation in the hospital in Iowa City. The first time was a shock, seeing her pale, splotchy and bloated. They had to dress up in booties and masks to keep the environment as sterile as possible. Back home, they lit a candle every day she was gone.

When asked if they ever considered that their mother might die, Maureen responds, "I don't think that dawned on me until after." When Diane returned, she adds that "Spending time together was one of the easiest things. We acted very normal."

Diane remembers having to take medication at noon every day

that would pretty much knock her out for a couple of hours. She'd take that nap on the sofa to be near her kids. "Just knowing the children were around was so comforting."

Kathleen says their relationship became stronger as the little things started to mean more. Part of her wanted someone to encourage her to talk, but that didn't happen. Diane said that was particularly gratifying that, while teens normally shy away, her kids grew closer. She calls herself the luckiest mom in the world for how intuitive, compassionate and responsible her children were and still are.

"I remember writing a paper at the end of my freshman year," Maureen says. "There was a lot more respect for my mom after seeing what she had been through and understanding how hard it must have been."

Teenagers can be selfish, but she realized she didn't want to be a burden on either of her parents, so she behaved, she says with a laugh. However, she wanted everything to get back to normal, for the medications and IV's to evaporate. They had to get rid of their dog, but they were more upset about the restrictions imposed on visitors because of germs.

At the younger end of the spectrum were Allen in fourth grade and Alison in sixth grade.

Alison didn't really understand what was going on, other than "things would be fine." She didn't know anyone who had had cancer or what it was all about. "I was scared at the time, but didn't fully understand the extent of what was going on. I could just brush it off."

> **Lesson #2**
> Kids can be embarrassed by all the focus on the sick parent

As the youngest, Allen didn't grasp the seriousness of the situation, other than his mom was sick. Diane's parents tried to reassure them, too, that it would be okay. He and Alison stuck closer together because of their closeness in age.

"When my mom was sick," he says, "she was not able to do everything with me like before. I felt like there was a major void in my life, which made me feel very sad, although I was relieved by my mom's positive attitude she always carried with her."

"I think my dad did a very good job keeping us involved in all of our activities," Alison says. "Things seemed pretty normal." People would ask about her, and she'd shrug it off. "I remember one time in sixth grade when everybody made cards for my mom. My teacher asked me to stand up and explain. I was so embarrassed. I didn't know what to say." She was also embarrassed when people were asked in church to pray for Diane.

"It was like a piece was missing in my life, but we did the same things, yet it didn't feel the same," Allen says. "She was always smiling, happy. 'So she's happy and doing okay.' "

He remembers her bald head and how shiny it was, and how they couldn't really hug her when she was in the hospital. He recalls her coming to one of his performances and how she sat in the back wearing a mask. "I didn't realize what a risk she was taking of getting sick by coming. She could have been exposed to all those germs."

Alison remembers their mom coming home for Christmas, how she had to go back that same night, and how her relatives were "freaking out." The kids also had to learn to keep the house a lot cleaner, she laughs, including all the rituals of washing their hands and not coming near her if they felt sick. It was odd when friends came over and having to make sure everybody washed their hands. She also remembers Diane walking around the house with her IV.

Alison learned more about cancer over time and finding out about other kids' experiences through Komen Kids, later Kids Konnected. They, too, realized how lucky they were. All of them except Allen went to California to learn about the program, and Alison laughingly admits, "I thought it was kind of dumb at first." Her enthusiasm increased as the program grew.

Allen agrees that it made it easier to talk to kids their own age, though he thought at the time the adults were "trapping" them into going to meetings because they went to fun places. Son and mother laugh in unison. It shows that just a hint of bribery does pay off to get kids talking without them even knowing they are.

"I was so shy," he says when asked if he talked to his mother privately. "I was so confused and didn't know what to ask."

Alison adds that "I don't think Dad ever hid anything from us. He let us know exactly what's going on. He'd tell us, 'Your mom isn't feeling well today' or whatever." She's still not sure if it would have been better to know then everything she now knows about the seriousness of the disease.

When they hear of someone they know who has cancer, they offer to talk and/or to listen, and share how they understand what someone is going through. Both agree that talking is an important way to get through it, reaching children at their appropriate maturity level. The younger ones thought the hair shaving ritual was fun along with Mom as Mr. Clean. The positive attitude did help them.

Since then, they've learned much about their mother's ordeal by the presentations she's given. When asked how they responded to her openness in discussing it publicly, Kathleen says it was a mixture of pride, the opening of old wounds, and quite emotional.

Maureen concurs. "There were times when it was like, 'I didn't know that,' hearing it for the first time like these strangers. I thought it was cool that she was so open to sharing it with them while secretly feeling guilty that I did not already know the information myself. However, I do realize that it has been and still is a learning process for her. It will be an ongoing learning process for her as she looks back at her life-threatening illness. In that way, I know that she might say something in a public speech in two years that she just realized the night before she gave the speech."

Kathleen says they probably wanted to forget their personal experience, "but it brought us closer, and we have a new appreciation for life. People need to hear her share her story and it inspires them. It's worth it to have some old wounds reopened." They credit their mother with bringing it to life because there were other children who had it a lot worse. In the beginning of the children's support group, they shared their experiences more for their mother than themselves, but also have been profoundly affected by it.

Maureen says parents and children must communicate what they're thinking. Kathleen wants to emphasize, "Don't have any regrets. Be sure you do and say everything you want." She's realized in recent years just how strong her mother was, and the ripple effect of her mom's illness and how many other people have been affected. Maureen says her mother evolved and became better at evaluating her priorities. "She wasn't afraid to make some changes."

Diane appreciated all the families and friends who pitched in to take care of her family and those individuals who gave the kids a little extra mothering. That's something other families can help with, offering rides or inviting the kids close to their children's ages to join in activities.

Lesson #3
Don't be afraid to step back and re-evaluate your life. Follow through & make changes if necessary.

"I communicate with the kids more now because I know things can change without notice. You want to let each other know how you feel," Diane says. "I'm lucky, lucky! I feel lucky looking back, even though I didn't feel so fortunate at the moment."

Children's common reactions to cancer

Parents and other adults may notice some of the following reactions in children facing the cancer of a loved one:

▶ Trying to help around the house
▶ Attempt to "be good"
▶ Giving more hugs and kisses
▶ Trying not to make any loud noises or disruptions in the house
▶ Becoming hypervigilent
▶ Begin to take over jobs of the survivor (cooking, cleaning, caring for younger children, etc)
▶ Acting out
▶ Poor grades in school
▶ Keeping up school grades so the parents have fewer worries
▶ Denial
▶ Regression in behavior
▶ Beginning to experiment with drugs and alcohol
▶ Confusion
▶ Becoming more active and staying away from the home
▶ Anger and rage
▶ Depression and the blues
▶ Isolation
▶ Asking a lot of questions
▶ Questioning God about the cancer
▶ Withdrawing into their "own world"
▶ Heightened anxiety
▶ Not wanting to bring friends to the house
▶ Guilt

The reactions of children and teens are individual and not all react in the same way. Encouraging your children to be part of a cancer support group, staying active in school and church activities, and having the warm support of family and friends will greatly assist in the type of reactions that manifest.

Helping children to cope eases everyone's transition

▶ *Learn the facts about cancer.* Eliminate myths such as believing that all forms of cancer are terminal, or the myth that if you have cancer it will always return.

▶ *Clarify to your child that they didn't give you cancer nor can they "catch" it from you.*

▶ *Teach children about the different types of feelings.* This gives children and teens the ability to name their feelings and discuss them.

▶ *Promote cancer education.* Explain the common terminology related to cancer, treatment, and diagnosis. Learn how cancer affects the body and how treatment modalities work to fight the cancer.

▶ *Talk about death in a free and open way.* If this is not relevant to your situation, then talk to your children about the fact that they do not need to worry about death. Trust us, it is a subject that needs to be discussed because your children will be thinking about it.

▶ *Help your children and teens learn forms of stress management.* Make sure they are active, eat nutritional meals and get plenty of sleep on a regular schedule.

▶ *Teach them communication techniques and effective ways to ask questions, as well as techniques for listening.*

▶ *Validate your children's and teen's experiences.* Remember, this is a family disease, and the cancer affects them, too.

▶ *Join a cancer support group for children or teens.*

▶ *Discuss topics in an age appropriate fashion.* Young preschoolers do not need to know as much detail as a pre-teen.

▶ *Work with your child to identify someone they trust who will be available to them when they have concerns.* Let them choose this person and develop an ongoing relationship with them.

▶ *Be open and honest.* This may be difficult but try to answer all the questions to the best of your knowledge.

▶ *Encourage your child to speak about their feelings with a licensed mental health counselor.*

▶ *Borrow from a local cancer center or library books that are specifically designed for children who have a parent with cancer.* There are many picture books available that show bald parents playing with their children, etc.

▶ *Ask your child to explain your cancer, treatment and prognosis.* This will give insight into any inaccurate information.

▶ *Create a cancer chore list.* Identify realistic and little things your child can do to be of assistance. Remember to note "fun things," too. Create a new routine together that is realistic for both of you, especially during treatment days. For example:
  • *Monday:* Pick up dirty clothes
  • *Tuesday:* Put dishes in dishwasher
  • *Wednesday:* Wear silly hats and watch a funny movie

▶ *If you anticipate a hospitalization, make arrangements to visit the unit prior to your stay.* Request a consultation with a child life specialist, staff counselor of social worker to explain hospital room equipment in an age and developmentally appropriate manner.

▶ *If your child requests to go to treatment with you, make arrangements with your cancer team prior to a scheduled treatment.* Also have a friend with you.

Cancer chore list

✏ _____

✏ _____

✏ _____

✏ _____

✏ _____

✏ _____

Survivors say...

9

What did your significant other do or say to assist you?

▶ She cared for me after surgery. For over a month cleaning and draining my hole in my back to allow healing from the inside out. *T, 69, skin*

▶ He said, "It could be a lot worse." *G, 81, uterine*

▶ The most wonderful man in the world! *T, 64, breast*

▶ He kept my spirits up. He told me how proud he was of my accepting my diagnosis and told me every day he loved me. *Marilyn, 72, breast*

▶ He did not mind my bald head. *Yvonne, 74, breast*

▶ Everything. He was my dearest friend. *Kathy, 61, breast*

▶ He was there for me 24 hours every day! *Maxine, 84, lung*

▶ He had Alzheimer's. Couldn't help. *N, 80, breast*

▶ Lived normally. *S, 61, breast*

▶ Nothing. Never. Very condescending. *C, 79, breast*

▶ Nothing. "We" died that day. *Diana, 46, lung*

▶ He never displayed negativity or fear in my presence. In some ways, acting like I just had the flu. Keeping things light. *Sandy, 58, breast*

▶ He gave wonderful back rubs. *Helen, 71, lymphoma*

▶ He was good about it, stuck with me, did whatever he could. *Betty, 68, breast*

▶ Concerned, but didn't know how to be supportive because he couldn't fix it. Need to be more knowledgeable for spouse to be compassionate. *L, 58, breast*

"He helped me focus on today, not what could happen in the future." Karen, 33, breast

▸ Unconditional love. He never acted embarrassed. *Rosalie, 80, breast*

▸ Support, that no matter what happens, I am still the same person. *V, 64, breast*

▸ He did not miss my breast at all. He was more loving, more caring. *Noor, 56, breast*

▸ Was very positive and was not concerned about the change in my body due to the mastectomy, that my health was most important to him. *Jude, 64, breast*

▸ Took care of me in ways he never dreamed he would be able to do. *Judy, 56, breast*

▸ My husband took me to each of my chemo treatments, but really wouldn't talk about how he felt or what he was thinking or didn't know. *Paula, 53, uterine and breast*

▸ Let me keep doing things. *Judy, 69, colon*

▸ Told me I was loved and needed. *V, 66, breast*

▸ My husband is my rock. He has given me his support and love. He is my knight in shining armor! *Elaine, 72, leukemia*

> "My wife said, 'Too many good things happened along the way. Must be a good reason for all of this. God is not going to let you die.'"
> Bill, 64, throat

▸ He died of cancer in 1998. I was his caregiver! *Donna, 72, colon*

▸ Praying together. Crying together, *Alveretta, 85, ovarian*

▸ Took me on little "tours" to help keep my mind off the pain. *Rita, 58, breast*

▸ I've been divorced 12 years. I was grateful he wasn't in my life when I was diagnosed and had surgery. He would have not been helpful! *Karen, 62, breast*

▸ He was there with constant hugs and assurances that everything would be fine, and we'd have a long life together. I needed to believe that. *Robin, 46, breast*

▸ I always got encouragement from my husband, but the most meaningful was when he cried with me. *Mary, 52, breast*

▶ I found dating one person in particular gave me energy, made me feel young again, but her departure halfway into treatment affected me negatively. *Joseph, 25, Hodgkin's lymphoma*

▶ Made me get up, take a shower every day, made me walk every day. Loved me. Tried to make me eat. *Helen, 72, lung*

▶ He said he loved me no matter how I might end up looking or feeling. He said I'm beautiful no matter what happens. *Martha, 51, breast*

▶ "You can beat this, we need you." *Okdoke, 67, uterine*

▶ I would wake my husband up in the night if I was afraid, and he would hold and comfort me. *Carolyn, 70, colon*

▶ "You're a tough little shit and you're going to make it!" *JoAnn, breast*

▶ I knew that he loved me no matter what. He's a little on the quiet side and in some ways I think it scared him more than it scared me. My staying positive helped him stay positive. *Ann, 45, breast*

▶ His father was going through cancer at the same time, so it was pretty rough. *Lori, 39, melanoma*

"Spouse of Survivor (SOS) was awesome about treating me as the person he married, not a victim or a fragile object that may break." Diane, 38, thyroid

"Things do not change; we change." Henry David Thoreau

Significant others: Ways to make me feel better

194

Cancer patients must remember how horribly stressful this is on their partners, and that in most cases, they are trying as hard as they can to help. It is very difficult for a partner to know the "right" thing to say or do, and there are no two survivors alike and what might be appreciated by one will not work for someone else.

Diane notes, "I am very lucky to have such a special spouse who has been very supportive and understanding of my life after breast cancer and a mastectomy. I was not fortunate enough to have had reconstruction and still have not 10 years after the initial surgery. My husband has made me feel complete without my right breast and has always been very sensitive about my surgery. Certainly it bothers me, but you would never know as he is so sensitive about it."

Use this list as a starting point. Circle items that you want or need on certain days. Also, ask them what they need or want to talk about. Together you are traveling this most difficult journey. These are what male and female survivors of various cancers have shared that they appreciate post-surgery:

▸ Tell me how much you love me — often!

▸ Ask me often if I would like to talk about "it."

▸ Make me feel as sexy and appreciated as I did before the surgery.

▸ Kiss the surgery site.

▸ I appreciate how you don't admire or discuss other women's attributes that I do not have.

▸ I love all the extra touching.

▸ I love to talk about our future together.

▸ I appreciate back rubs and foot rubs.

▸ I appreciate your sensitivity to when I need some "alone" time and know that it is not you.

▸ Understand when I need extra family and friends time.

▸ Ask what special dinner I would like and could you make it for me.

▸ Take me out for dinner.

- Don't be afraid to be intimate as we were before and ask me what I would like.
- Take me out to do my favorite hobby.
- Don't compare me to other cancer patients who recovered faster, better, etc.
- Don't discuss other individuals who may not have made it and how it was a "blessing" due to their condition.

195

- Dote on me.
- Tell me what you can do to help me through this.
- Communicate with me so we can be closer than ever.
- Help me enjoy intimacy like never before.
- Touch my face.
- Rub my head.
- Wink at me.
- Go with me to all my doctors' appointments.
- Say how wonderful I look without my wig on.
- Read to me when I am too sick to read myself.
- Make me laugh.
- Pump me up when I'm down.
- Tell me I am the most handsome/beautiful special partner you have ever seen.
- Give me lots of compliments.
- Help me be strong.
- Take me to a movie.
- Help me pretend occasionally to escape from this terrible disease.
- Look at me in the same adoring way when we first met.
- Tell the doctor whatever it takes for my treatment to be successful no matter what.
- Tell me that you will always be here for me.
- I appreciate it when you brag about me to your friends and co-workers about how brave and special I am.
- I need you to put cool cloths on my head as I am so uncomfortable after chemo.
- Please just sit by me and be my best friend. Knowing you are there is the most comforting thought.

Loved ones offer advice to others

196

Our family and friends also put together some ideas that they found helpful to assist in their journey with their loved one. The following are their suggestions to other friends and family members:

▸ Don't give up
▸ Organize an aggressive plan of attack
▸ Listen
▸ Give the person space, and don't smother them
▸ Maintain a sense of humor
▸ Be patient
▸ Be kind to each other
▸ Show your love and appreciation
▸ Stay positive
▸ Encourage and support your survivor
▸ Do exactly what the doctors say
▸ Go with them to all appointments
▸ Take notes at medical appointments
▸ Help monitor appropriate visiting and calling times for your loved one's friends
▸ Join a support group
▸ Get educated on the specific cancer and treatment
▸ Accept help from others
▸ Stay physically close to the survivor
▸ Do something special for your loved one a few times a week
▸ Explore alternative treatment options for them
▸ Talk about death and arrangements
▸ Consider quality of life over quantity
▸ Don't take one minute for granted
▸ Stay mentally and physically in good shape
▸ Share feelings with each other
▸ Do not feel guilty to take time off for yourself
▸ Always get a second opinion
▸ Establish an information phone and e-mail chain for all of their concerned friends
▸ Be available
▸ Be honest
▸ Smile a lot

- Keep the lines of communication open with your loved one
- Don't take your loved one's frustration or depression personally
- Choose a hospital based on good recommendations from other patients/families
- Talk about the illness
- Encourage others to visit for short periods
- Let the survivor have the deciding vote on the treatment
- Help your loved one feel useful and valued by asking for their opinions
- Talk about happy memories
- Ask doctors lots of questions and be an advocate
- Be aware of changes in the survivor and keep records of them

- Accept the situation
- Support their entire family
- Be assertive with hospital care
- Become financially educated
- Help your loved one stay clean and groomed
- Keep living your life
- Write down your feelings and tape record conversations
- Treat your loved one as normal as possible
- Stay strong
- Call the American Cancer Society, St. Jude or similar cancer group for a listing of services in your area
- Pray
- Remember that silence is okay
- Respect their wishes
- Do not tell them about every new treatment you read about

197

Top responses

- ✎ Stay physically close to them
- ✎ Show love and appreciation
- ✎ Encourage and support
- ✎ Give them space & don't smother
- ✎ Stay positive

Loved ones say...

Based on your experience, what would you now recommend to other caregivers, loved ones or friends?

▶ Don't let the cancer diagnosis take over your life. Look at how to *live* life with it as an inconvenience. *Laura, 44, father, prostate*

▶ Be a good listener. Give the patient emotional space. Don't smother them. *Doug, 57, wife, breast*

▶ Do not give in. When you are planning treatments and have a plan of attack, it helps rather than giving up. It helped both mentally and physically to have several good years, feeling good, too. *L, 66, husband, prostrate*

▶ Let the patient have more input in how he wants treatment. And talk openly about death. Encourage people to visit him for short periods. *Colleen, 60, husband, colon*

▶ Acknowledge the fear, push through it and talk about what is happening. *Julie, 51, father, lung*

▶ Attitude is the most important thing. Smile. Know you are both in this awful thing together and let them know you believe life goes on and it will not hurt either of you. *Marianne, 71, husband, large cell lymphoma*

▶ Get them to realize they need to get actively engaged in their care and the responsibility of their disease rather than ignore it and leave the care/responsibility to others and doctors. *Judith, 70, husband, colon*

▶ Stay close, support and understand the times of frustration and depression. *John, 55, wife, breast*

▶ Get past issues out in the open and deal with current issues as they arise. Keep faith and welcome friends. *Bette, 57, husband, melanoma*

▶ Communicate more and don't worry about becoming emotional. *Martha, 50, mother, non-Hodgkins lymphoma*

▶ Be honest, smile, believe, stay positive. *Georgia, 48, father, lung*

▶ Be there when you can and step away when it gets heavy and don't feel guilty about "down time" you need. *Mary, 42, father, lung*

▶ Talk to your doctor and see if there is medication or other treatments to keep the caregiver as normal and in as good health as possible. *Darrell, 54, wife, lung*

▶ I still meet regularly with the three women from my widows' support group. Talk about death and expectations. Don't try everything the doctors recommend. Consider quality of life over quantity. Take care of your own health. Be realistic and truthful with your kids according to their age to accept. Realize that expressions of grief change, and it lasts a *lot* longer than you or anyone else expects. Other people *don't* always know how you're feeling, but show appreciation for any attempts. *Mary, 52, husband, kidney*

199

▶ Every minute is precious. Don't take your friends or relatives for granted. Encourage them. Look for positive things. Don't overlook a sunrise, flowers, a bird, a new snowfall. *Kathleen, 49, friend, breast*

▶ Do every little thing you can think of to bring even just a small amount of joy to the person. I had my mom's grandfather clock fixed, and she enjoyed it during her last days. *Tracy, 47, mother, lung*

"Be kind to each other and express gratitude for her contribution to our relationship." *Rudy, 81, wife, leukemia*

▶ Know that being close without having to say or do anything is sometimes what's needed and appreciated. *Laura, 44, aunt, lymph*

▶ Be patient, listen to all feelings, concerns and be aware of all the different emotions they are experiencing. *Wayne, 48, wife, breast*

▶ Listen to your gut. If you feel that something's wrong with yourself, spouse or whomever, it probably is. Get competent medical help immediately. *Linda, 62, husband, colon*

▶ Offer hope and love. Support the whole family, not just the person with cancer. No matter the outcome, use the insights this ordeal gives you to be a better person. *Monica, 35, husband, pancreatic*

▶ Express your feelings. Show that you care. Be "physical." *Shirley, 66, brother, lung*

▶ Be as patient and understanding as possible. Pray, pray, pray. Make the most of every day. *Lisa, 40, husband, brain*

▸ Listen with your heart and break all the rules. *Mary, 63, best friend, breast*

▸ You know the person best. *Liz, 43, sister, breast*

▸ Look to other sources to share your pain and frustrations of watching someone you love suffer. Take time to walk, go to a movie, go on a date, cry often, laugh a lot. *Rue, 29, mother, breast*

▸ Love them, listen to them. They just want to be treated like they always were. Be positive. *Patti, 52, husband, kidney*

▸ Be there to show your love and encouragement. Be strong and stay positive. Tell them that you love them and show it. *Randy, 46, wife, breast*

▸ Make sure the patient knows making a meal or giving small gifts makes the caregiver feel better. It's hard not to be able to do anything when you want to help. *Diane, 38, friend/co-worker, breast*

▸ To be up front with the person and find out as much information as possible. *Krista, 39, father, prostate*

▸ Be a positive supporter. Help by learning about the treatments available and provide the patient with the encouragement that those treatments will be effective. *Gerald, 67, wife, breast*

▸ Don't be afraid to get close if it feels right to all involved. Respect each other's experience and perspective (patient, caregiver, spouse, child). Use available resources for knowledge. Don't be "too strong." *Ann, 51, friend, brain*

▸ Support their decisions, whether they are "yours" or not. *N, 68, friend, breast*

▸ We let the patient and family know we were praying for them and thinking of them, and that we were available for help if wanted or needed. And if they did ask, we made sure we would be there to provide it. *Roger, 56, and Char, 59, friend, prostate*

▸ Let other people help you. They want to help. Pray and pray. God listens. Don't tell the patient about some cure you read about. You may do as much harm as help. *Chuck, 61, wife, rectal*

▸ Open up and talk. Ask the questions that only that person can answer before it's too late. *Chris, 38, mother, breast*

▸ Give your patient all the love and support you can. Talk to them, visit them. Push them when they need it, but respect and accept their decisions. Let them know you love them. *Mark, 45, wife, breast*

▸ You don't have to say much. Just be strong and be there to hug and listen. *Mike, 56, wife, tongue*

▸ Be as supportive as possible, read key pieces of information on diagnosis. Communications with doctors is vital, ask lots of questions, solicit support from family/friends. *Mary, 48, husband, thyroid*

▸ Shower them with love and don't get angry about petty things. *Kathleen, 24, mother, breast*

▸ Keep communication open and don't assume you know how they feel. *David, 67, wife, breast*

▸ Just be there for them in whatever capacity. To help care for them or just listen to them or sit with them. But always treat them normally. Because even though they might not feel normal, they are. *Barb, 44, best friend, non-Hodgkins lymphoma*

▸ Respect their wishes as far as privacy. Let them know that you are there, but don't push. Let them call the shots. There are times when they want to be down, so let them. *Monica, 52, sister, NA*

▸ Don't be afraid to offer to do fun things as well, but don't assume practical things are being taken care of. *Sharon, 65, friend, breast*

▸ Help the patient work through stages on their schedule. Don't downplay. Don't say everything will be all right unless you are 100 percent sure. *Peggy, 53, husband, prostate*

"I knew how my life would change. At first she looked treatable, and there wasn't a huge concern. I did have thoughts that it would reoccur. I told her that I was going to always think the worst before each doctor's appointment, and then things could only be better. That way we couldn't be overwhelmed, or they couldn't say anything that was worse than what we created in our minds. It was my coping mechanism. I admit it." L, wife, breast

I love you

Sometimes our survivors feel like the cancer has "stolen" the essence of who they are. Friends and loved ones can help survivors stay positive by reminding them of their positives. Or perhaps, the survivor can use positives to remind their loved ones how much they love and appreciate them. Here are some ideas to get you going.

What I love about you

❑ Your smile

❑ The sound of your laughter

❑ The color of your eyes

❑ The way you tell me you love me

❑ Your warm hugs

❑ The way you treat me

❑ Your strength and perseverance

❑ Your sense of humor

❑ Your creativity

❑ Your effort

❑ _____

❑ _____

❑ _____

❑ _____

❑ _____

Be prepared for some changes

Cancer is a devastating state of adversity for a relationship. It has the potential to tear the relationship to shreds, or it has the potential to intensify the strength and love of those involved. Adversity can create a crisis or it can be an opportunity. The choice is yours … it is all in the way in which you choose to treat the adversity. You have the power to find the lessons within the trauma.

Cancer does change lives … but it also has the ability to bring loved ones closer. Our survey illustrates that some significant others see some negative or diminishing factors in their relationships, but for the most part, our survivors see this adversity that they shared as an opportunity for growth, compassion, and enhancements for their relationship. Those who found a "life lesson" also discovered a purpose, meaning or something to make them feel grateful. They learned ways to overcome the adversity.

> "Embrace change even though the timing could not be more difficult."
> Diane, 47, breast

How significant others viewed changes

Here's how our significant others believe their relationship with their survivor changed due to the diagnosis of cancer:

- ▶ We openly discuss our feelings now
- ▶ We have a more caring relationship
- ▶ We are closer as a couple
- ▶ We've learned to communicate better
- ▶ We've learned to value each day
- ▶ Our relationship did not change at all, or very little
- ▶ We now have a deeper love for each other

- I became the parent instead of the spouse
- Our friendship became adult/child relationship
- I became the parent instead of the child
- I became the older sister instead of the younger one
- Our faith was strengthened
- I'm now more protective of my loved one
- Our sexual relationship was heightened, and we became more physical
- I now have more respect for my loved one
- We now have more honesty in our relationship
- I now value my significant other more
- Our sexual relationship became nonexistent
- My loved one communicated less and became more closed off
- We became more considerate of each other
- We seem to understand each other more
- We became more dependent on each other
- It became a more stressful and overwhelming relationship
- We became more sensitive to each other's needs

Top responses

- We are closer as a couple
- Little or no change
- We value each other more
- We now have a deeper love for each other
- I became the parent instead of the spouse

Loved ones say...

How did your relationship with the individual change?

▶ My dad has opened up to me more. *Laura, 44, father, prostate*

▶ Value each day we have together. *Doug, 57, wife, breast*

▶ We were always close, but we became closer. *L, 66, husband, prostrate*

▶ Saw each other more frequently, took family vacation. *Julie, 51, father, lung*

▶ Less intimacy. He somewhat pulled away, less outwardly loving. *Virginia, 66, husband, colon; mother-in-law, colon*

▶ I had more of a "mothering " attitude toward him. *Judith, 70, husband, colon*

▶ We got closer and relied on each other more. *John, 55, wife, breast*

▶ Angry that she would not talk to us about what she was going through. *James, 55, mother, colon*

▶ He became more alive and made comments like, "We should walk, it's a beautiful day! There will never be another day like this one!" *Bette, 57, husband, melanoma*

▶ It changed drastically. I paid 100 percent attention to her and tried to give her comfort. *Rosemary, 66, sister, ovarian*

▶ I had to take responsibility for everything. *P, 62, husband, throat and neck*

▶ The stay in the ICU changed us by bringing us closer. *Darrell, 54, wife, lung*

▶ No intimacy. *Rudy, 81, wife, leukemia*

▶ For the first year, we were extremely close. As he progressed further into remission, he got back to his "same old self," worrying about money, house cleaning, trivial things. *Patti, 52, husband, kidney*

▶ Became more spiritual. Little stuff didn't matter as much, more honest. *Mary, 52, husband, kidney*

▶ My sister and I became the caregivers. My mother was an unselfish caregiver all her life raising 10 children, being a devoted mother. *L, 50, mother, lung*

▶ Never did. I loved them before, during and after. *Vera, 73, several relatives*

▶ I became the mother, and he became the child. *Bertha, 84, husband, prostate*

▶ I became more the caretaker of a "child" than a wife and lover. Verbal communication is almost non-existent. *Pat, 57, husband, brain*

▶ I felt very hurt and shut out of his life for the first time in over 35 years of marriage. *Linda, 62, husband, colon*

▶ I respected him more because of the innerstrength he exhibited. *Abbie, 51, father, leukemia*

▶ We continued to be very close. He tried to give me a hard time at times, but I thought he just didn't feel well. *Lynn, 64, brother, colon*

▶ We were both more loving, more considerate of each other. I always thought the kids were the priority, and we'd have more time together when they were older. This changed, and he became my number one priority. *Monica, 35, husband, pancreatic*

▶ We became closer. He expressed his feelings for the first time since becoming an adult. I became very protective and solicitous. *Shirley, 66, brother, lung*

▶ We became closer emotionally. I could "read" Mom better than before. *Rue, 29, mother, breast*

> "My mom has always been the strongest person I had ever known. After her diagnosis, she seemed so much weaker and needy." *Carlene, 51, mother, breast*

▶ We are even closer now. I now know that my wife is the most important thing in my life. *Bill, 59, wife, breast*

▶ For the best, she is sexier and making up for lost time. *Ron, 62, wife, breast*

▸ I could do for her instead of her always doing for me. *Kay, 65, mother, leukemia*

▸ At first, it did not change. Toward the end, I was not only a spouse but the sole caregiver as to a child in need. *Leonard, 41, wife, breast*

▸ To deeper friendship, more accepting of "Yes, it could happen to me or anybody" for both of us. *Ann, 51, friend, brain*

▸ We are closer. I've had breast cancer also. *Bambi, 47, mother and sister, breast*

▸ I love and appreciate our time spent together more than ever. *Beverly, 50, best friend, mesothelioma*

▸ Closer and more sharing of feelings. Priorities of my time and hers changed. Each day has been a gift, not 24 hours to get through. *Pam, friend, breast and lung*

▸ We got closer as the illness progressed. We also kept our work relationship alive with a lot of mentoring, even over the phone. *Diane, 38, friend/co-worker, breast*

▸ Our relationship has always been deep. An experience like this only deepened our love for each other. It also made our attitudes change toward living. "Why put off tomorrow" kind of attitude. We live for today. *Mary, 48, husband, thyroid*

▸ I respected his strength and courage. *C, 63, father, esophageal and liver*

▸ Became more aware of how much I cared about her and vice versa. *Kathleen, 24, mother, breast*

▸ We became one in our battle against cancer, like soldiers. But inside my other identity was dealing with increasingly being a single parent, under financial strain, pressures at work (missed time). I was becoming isolated. And yet, my sole purpose for living was to keep her alive. *Paul 53, wife, breast*

▸ She was a strong person who remained the mother until she died. *Nancy, 67, mother, pancreatic*

▸ Had to watch the clock more. We made the time matter. *Michael, 50, wife*

▸ He was a very proud man. His feelings were kept deep inside of him. *Jeanne, 53, father, liver*

Survivors reveal emotions

Our survey opened the door for survivors who had been repressing many of their emotions. We were struck by the intensity and diversity of the responses as it related to how cancer had affected their relationships with their significant others and friends.

These results might be startling to you. Many of our survivors believe they are surviving *because* of the love and compassionate actions of their loved ones. Love and affiliation do help us be resilient and give us strength to endure what we may not have thought we could face.

You will also learn the secret thoughts and feelings of those who have many times suffered in silence. Holding in their pain and resentment, many survivors grieve the loss of support, empathy, compassion, nurturing, and caring from their significant others and friends.

How did cancer affect your relationships?

- Discovered I wasn't alone
- The cancer brought me closer to my husband
- My husband couldn't look at me without my breast
- My friends drifted away
- My life is now more spontaneous
- Today I'm more willing to travel and enjoy my life to the fullest
- The cancer brought me closer to all my friends
- The cancer brought me closer to God
- People in my life became distant
- My daughter wouldn't accept my diagnosis and the reality of my limitations
- My family would not join a support group, and this was very disheartening
- The cancer brought me closer to those I love
- My family ignored my situation
- My spouse ignored my situation
- My husband showed a lack of compassion for my needs
- The cancer affected our sexual relationship
- Now I appreciate life and each person in my life
- My friendships are reinforced and filled with new friends

- Today I am closer to my children
- Cancer may be the major cause of my divorce
- My feelings were hurt because some friends didn't bother to call or even send a card
- Some family members just stayed away, there was no contact at all, and they just couldn't handle it
- Family and friends were amazed at my positive attitude
- My marriage sucks. My husband is retired and gone most of the day, and I'm all alone
- Now I'm conscious of the fragility of life
- Friends just dropped out of my life
- This taught me to do things instead of putting them off
- Three of my friends left me because they didn't believe I should have dark days
- Now I'm a more compassionate person
- People apologized after my treatment for not being there for me
- I'm separated from my husband now because he couldn't cope with the reality of what was happening
- My friends were scared and I found myself making sure I looked healthy and acted like I was feeling well. I think this put a huge strain on me
- One of my closest friends couldn't deal with my cancer
- I decided not to want to see some people who could not be connected as friends — life is too short for that
- I had a mastectomy and I'm so embarrassed about the way I look

209

Top responses

🖉 My husband was not supportive
🖉 My friends were not supportive
🖉 The cancer brought us closer
🖉 My friends pulled away
🖉 My spouse pulled away

210

How would I like my relationship to be with my loved ones?

_____

_____

_____

_____

_____

_____

_____

_____

_____

_____

_____

_____

Survivors say...

How did cancer affect your relationships?

- It strengthened my husband's and my relationship. Time is short. You don't know what tomorrow will bring. *Tracy, 33, cervical*

- My husband was perhaps not helpful enough with household help. Maybe he was in denial? *Judith, 70, breast*

- They are stronger. My husband of 53 years and I are closer and more in love than before. Friends and neighbors are more open and so caring. *Elaine, 72, leukemia*

- My friends didn't call or come to see me, save three people. Everyone had their hands full and no time. Only good intentions. *Donna, 72, colon*

- My husband was more loving. He loves me and not my body. He is more caring after the cancer than before. *Noor, 56, breast*

- Everyone stayed very positive and friends and family worried, but stayed about the same. They know I'm a survivor. *Maria, 61, breast*

- Friendships were reinforced, and new friends were made on this journey that will last a lifetime. You truly realize what it means to call someone "your friend." *Paula, 53, uterine, breast*

- I am not so future-focused. I am much more focused on the present. More spontaneous, seeking new experiences and willing to spend available money to travel and enjoy life. Others find this change a little disconcerting. *Jim, 50, thyroid*

- Made them stronger. *John 81, prostate and colon*

- No sexual relations because of fear I would be hurt. My job was dropped. I worked there 11 years and nobody cared. *Karen, 51, lung*

- I maintained a positive attitude, which helped them. *B, 93, breast*

- I think everybody handled it pretty well. *Betty, 68, breast*

- I haven't quite figured that one out yet. *Jennifer, 42, breast*

212

▶ Since I was not married at the time and not dating either, I was then and still am concerned how I could explain and be open to significant others. My cancer has probably kept me from pursuing an intimate relationship with someone because I don't know how to go about it. I know it shouldn't be important, but I'm concerned that it would be, probably more to me than him. *Mary, 64, breast*

▶ With my husband, more open communication, more reliance on each other. *Karen, 33, breast*

▶ Strengthened them. We realized our own mortalities and value each and every day and each and every person. Take nothing for granted and appreciate life and everyone. *Judy, 56, breast*

"My husband could not look at me, where the breast had been removed." *Loretta, 84, breast*

▶ We're a close family, always there for each other. This helps when something like this hits. *Betty, 74, NA*

▶ I didn't have the sex drive I'd had. I didn't want my husband to see me, but that was only one-sided. *Rosalie, 80, breast*

▶ Just my brother and sister-in-law, but they had their own health problems. *Dona, 74, NA*

▶ The only effect I have noticed is it brought me closer to those I love. *Sandy, 58, breast*

▶ Probably the cancer made me and my children more conscious of the frailty of life and how precious it is. *Marilyn, 70, adenoid cystic carcinoma*

▶ This experience strengthened my marriage and made me realize that not too much in life is that important to worry about. Like my mom always said, "If you have your health, you have everything." *Mary, 52, breast*

▶ I guess I am lucky. Life is pretty much the same. We don't dwell on possible recurrence. People are still praying for me and inquire, "How are you feeling?" *Jude, 64, breast*

▶ People became more distant. My pastor really cared. *C, 79, breast*

▶ It did not affect anything because I wouldn't let it! *Patricia, 73, breast*

▶ There was really no change. I would have liked to have a healthy husband around for the support. *Betty, 75, breast*

▶ We were both cancer patients. Our calendar revolved around doctors appointments, radiation, chemo, etc. *V, 66, breast*

▶ My husband, much deeper love and appreciation for our life. My mom and kids, we know we can count on each other. Friends? No one really asks about it, and we don't discuss. *Robin, 46, breast*

213

▶ My son and daughter-in-law were so quick to be available. I hadn't realized how much I could count on them. My brother was wonderful also. I'll never forget his being so constantly in touch. *Karen, 62,* breast

▶ Their love and support were terrific. Made us all aware of how great life is. *Judy, 69, colon*

▶ Some family members just stayed away, no contact at all. They just couldn't handle what they saw as my cancer treatment went on, the loss of weight and all my hair, my overall illness and chemotherapy. *Alveretta, 85, ovarian*

▶ Daughter will not face reality about how sick I've been and my limitations. Lives 30 miles away and comes twice a month. She does work. Has never gone to treatment with me. *Dorothy, 70, breast*

▶ I saw them all differently. My focus changed. Much closer to my children. May have been the major cause of divorce. Stress induced loss of testosterone levels, came back with treatment. *Robert, 70, lung*

▶ I hate my husband's lack of compassion for my needs. He continued social events without me and went away for six weeks. Telling me not to call, he would call me. Denial. *L, 58, breast*

▶ My relationship with family and friends became better and better. Their support was beyond price. *Mary, 62, breast*

> " My niece lives with us, and she is wonderful to me. Makes me laugh often." *Kathy, 61, breast*

▶ I have a deeper appreciation for my family and friends, neighbors. People are wonderful! *Mary Ann, 56, colon*

▶ My husband was not really supportive or understanding. Daughter helped by just being there. Friends and co-workers surprised me by sending flowers, cards, meals, calling. I found out I wasn't alone. *Theresa, 49, breast*

▶ I got out of shape and osteoarthritis snuck in, put on a lot of weight and am not (so far) able to get it off. My marriage sucks. My husband is retired and gone most of the time, and I'm alone. *Rita, 58, breast*

"Some of my friends kind of drifted away." Murray, 64, lymphoma

▶ I tried to stay the course and be like before. I didn't fake being positive, and I don't think I was real negative. *Bill, 64, throat, tongue*

▶ I was very alone. My mother was the only source of compassion, but there was very little she could do. People seemed to think the way to deal with it was to express nothing to me. *Joseph, 25, Hodgkin's lymphoma*

▶ Some people stay away. Some come nearer and become better friends. *Martha, 51, breast*

▶ It created the realization of the love and compassion of family and friends, which I sometimes ignore or forget how important they are to me. *Janet, 65, breast*

▶ I feel that I've grown and become more confident. My husband and I grew even closer. It helped us two years later to get through a difficult situation. *Barbara, 48, breast*

▶ I felt very vulnerable and very dependent during the time surrounding my diagnosis and surgery. There were some people that I didn't even tell because I did not wish to discuss things with them. You want some privacy. *Julie, 61, breast*

▶ I have a good friend that won't accept my recurrence the second time around. She shies away from me and won't talk about the "C" word. *Norma, 56, mesothelomia*

▶ I now have family members that can say "I love you" and give me a hug, show those feelings that were never outwardly expressed. More phone calls and visits from out-of-town family. Sit with friends, do nothing and realize that it is priceless. *Sara, 35, lung*

▸ I am very guarded in the way I spend my time. I try to not let other people plan my life. I don't like to be with people who make me uncomfortable. I like to be with people who truly love me for who I am and come away feeling good about the time I spent with them. *Noreen, 49, breast*

▸ You find out who your real friends are. *Christine, 51, breast*

▸ I saw how much my family really loved me. I knew they did, but in situations like this, there is nothing like a wonderful family to help you through. My 15-year-old daughter had a very rough time with it. It was like she was mad at me the entire time. Now that all my treatments are done, and she saw that I'm a survivor, we are closer than ever. *Melinda, 46, breast*

▸ It brought the whole family closer, except for one child, but he had a hard time dealing with the whole thing. Years later it is a lot better, but if a certain test comes up, the one child is still very quiet. *Carol, 71, colon*

▸ My family is closer. It is sad to say, but most of the friends I had I no longer have as friends, just because the outlook on life for me is a lot different than theirs. *Ana, 35, breast*

▸ Cancer makes me speak my mind, advocate for others. Sharing stories, fears and opinions is healing. *Diane, 38, thyroid*

▸ Most of my relationships got better and continue to grow in depth. It's an experience that you cannot ignore. *Ann, 45, breast*

"My husband had and still has a hard talking about it. I think my friends just became more grateful for their good health and loved life more." A survivor

Friendship bonds

- ▶ Listening, listening, listening. They need to share feelings, plans, thoughts. *Pam, friend, breast and lung*

- ▶ I think letting her know she was still important and needed at work helped her know she was a legacy (would be) and her expertise will always be needed. *Diane, 38, friend/co-worker, breast*

- ▶ We had some strange phone chats and she could talk about physical and emotional problems with me and not be embarrassed. We laughed a lot, too! *Susan, 49, best friend, lymphoma*

- ▶ Our friendship grew stronger. I think she counted on her friends to be with her and to help her, and this gave her peace, a sense she would not be left alone. *Sharon, 65, friend, breast*

- ▶ Praying for her, reading scriptures, listening, writing notes, encouraging words, continuing to share with her my life situations and allowing her to show her care, too. *Kathleen, 49, friend, breast*

A friend's hidden pain

When Norma was diagnosed with mesothelomia, which required the removal of her right lung, she was surprised when a close friend seemed to abandon her. This friend would back away whenever Norma mentioned the cancer, and this behavior troubled Norma.

It would be a year later before she would discover the reason why her friend had turned away. The answer came in an apologetic e-mail, how sorry she was that she hadn't been there for Norma. This woman's father had died of cancer, and she had known other people who had also died from this disease. Hearing Norma's news had brought all those bad and painful memories to the forefront, making her relive it all over.

What was even more telling was the friend's admission that she hadn't known anyone who had survived cancer. Sympathizing with her friend's very real fears, Norma had the perfect response:

"You do now."

Mental health & beyond

"Fear less, hope more;
Whine less, breathe more;
Talk less, say more;
Hate less, love more;
And all good things are
yours." Swedish proverb

What really matters in life?

Here's an exercise to help you assess what really is important and valuable in your life. Try this experiment:

▶ Name the five wealthiest people in the world.
▶ Name the last five winners of the NBA tournament
▶ Name the last five winners of the Miss America contest.
▶ Name five people who have won the Nobel Peace prize
▶ Name the last half dozen Academy Award winners for best actor and actress.
▶ Name the last five World Series winners.

How did you do? We bet you didn't know the greatest majority of the answers.

Now let's try part two of this experiment. Write your responses on the facing page. See how you do on this one:

▶ List two teachers who aided your journey through school.
▶ Name three friends who have helped you through this difficult time.
▶ Name five people who have taught you something worthwhile.
▶ Think of two loved ones who have been encouraging and supportive.
▶ Think of five people you enjoy spending time with.
▶ Name some survivors whose stories have inspired you.

We bet the second experiment was much easier for you to accomplish. So what's the lesson? The people who make a difference in your life are not the ones who have made the most money, who have won an Oscar, or have a championship ring. No, the people who really matter are the ones who have been there to help us through good times, bad times, and everything in between.

Love, friendship and connections are what really matter in our lives.

Who matters to me!

List two teachers who aided my journey through school

_____   _____

Name three friends who have helped me through this difficult time

_____   _____

_____

Name five people who have taught me something worthwhile.

_____   _____

_____   _____

_____

Think of two loved ones who have been encouraging and supportive

_____   _____

Think of five people you enjoy spending time with

_____   _____

_____   _____

_____

Name some survivors whose stories have inspired me

_____   _____

_____   _____

Bonus: Name members of my medical team who have been helpful or displayed compassion towards me

_____   _____

_____   _____

Good self-esteem is an important part of coping with cancer

220

It's hard to define, but easy to know if you have it or not. Self-esteem is generally viewed as a positive attitude about one's self. It is the ability to believe in our abilities and see ourselves as competent, in control, and capable. Unfortunately, too many of us believe we lack the confidence to become all that we desire.

Oprah is quoted as saying, "Each of us arrives with all we need to feel valued and unique, but slowly that gets chipped away … One life event after another can change our perception of who we are: rejection, divorce, or job loss leave us feeling not pretty enough, not good enough, not smart enough." But self-esteem is something we can nurture and build upon, creating a better sense of self.

Do you wonder where your low self-esteem originated? Family relationships are many times considered the determining factor in positive self-esteem. Parents play a vital role in nurturing and encouraging the development of self-confidence and positive regard. Simple techniques of praising and witnessing accomplishments may seem trite, but they are the soil for growing positive self-esteem. Achievements in childhood, which are reinforced, create self-confidence and belief in one's ability to interact within their environment. Many children also develop self-confidence when they learn skills to cope with difficult tasks or situations. These positive achievements promote belief in one's abilities and strengthen our belief in managing our internal stressors.

As part of my workshops (Miller) on self-esteem, I divide the group into "partners" and ask them to play the "apples and oranges game." This game is nothing more than an exercise in self-esteem. Each person is asked to spend a minimum of three minutes listing their own positive traits. As you can imagine, after about one minute most people run out of things to say. Pushed to continue, the participants are forced to keep the litany of positive statements going for over five minutes. Sadly, the participants note how difficult the task actually became during the time period. Most participants say they could have easily filled five minutes with all of their negatives but had difficulty acknowledging their positives. Unfortunately, our culture has taught us to acknowledge our negatives, but has not reinforced the powerful need to promote self-regard.

Positive self-esteem can be cultivated. People with high self-esteem appear to believe in themselves; in fact they appear to have self-respect.

This explains self-esteem in general. What we must remember is that cancer patients/survivors and other individuals who battle serious health concerns face a unique challenge in retaining or rebuilding their self-esteem. They may have to factor in chemo or radiation, weight gain or loss, constant flu-like symptoms, hair loss and the basic fight for their lives. All these are obstacles that have to be conquered in addition to everyday life. Keep that in mind when being around a survivor as they rebuild themselves emotionally and physically.

What are some of the basic building blocks for creating positive self-esteem, no matter who you are?

▶ *Individuality:* Appreciate your uniqueness, the traits that make you special. It may sound corny, but it is valuable to make a list of the unique positive attributes that you possess. How can anyone else appreciate or respect you, when you don't see your own positive qualities?

▶ *Integrity:* Know what you value and live accordingly. Make choices that are consistent with your values, morals, and beliefs. When we have integrity and a foundation for our life, we can trust ourselves and become more competent and self-respecting.

▶ *Connection:* Make connections with others that are intimate, strong, and supportive. The healthy connection with others boosts our belief in our worthiness and esteem. Each of us can enhance our self-esteem by developing healthy relationships with others, but most importantly by developing a healthy relationship with ourselves.

▶ *Personal power:* Believe that you can make changes, affect things in a positive way. Look around you and see the changes you have created. Look at what things you accomplish each and every day and reinforce all that you do. Confidence is built on seeing our own value and acknowledging the powerful force that we hold within.

▶ *Risk-taking:* Take chances and persevere despite failures or setbacks. Those with positive self-regard see failures and mistakes as opportunities for growth. Reward yourself for taking risks and for stretching beyond your comfort zone. A cancer diagnosis mandates that you take risks. It thrusts you far beyond that warm comfort zone. Confidence is gained as you realize you can accomplish things you never thought possible. So give yourself credit where credit is due.

▸ *Achievement:* Recognize your accomplishments, no matter how small. Set attainable goals to create pride in yourself.

▸ *Self-respect:* Believe that you are a good person, that you have abilities and talents that are worthwhile. Part of self-respect is also a belief that you deserve to be treated in a positive fashion by others (as well as yourself).

Self-esteem and self-confidence have a lot to do with your mental well-being and your ability to heal. If you want to change, and seek that change, it will occur. Your most powerful technique is seeing your potential and making changes to acknowledge your purpose, your achievements, and your value and uniqueness.

The real truth about stress

We all have it, each and every day of our lives, but do we really understand it? Let's take a look at some of the common myths related to stress in an effort to better deal with the stressors that sometimes tie us in knots.

▸ *Is stress always something bad for you?* Let's compare stress to a guitar string. When there is not enough tension the guitar sounds dull and twangy. If the string is too tight, the guitar sounds shrill or it might even snap. Stress is quite similar: If we have it in perfect balance, stress can be a motivator to make positive changes in our life. But, if we are out of balance, stress can cause us to become out of alignment. It is all in the way we learn to work with our stress.

▸ *If you are not having any physical symptoms, does that mean there is no stress in your life?* The absence of stress doesn't mean you aren't experiencing stress. Many people have successfully blocked their awareness of symptoms, while others may be using medication to block the signals. Sometimes a headache, stomach ache, back pain or stomach acid can be a warning sign of stressors in your life.

222

▶ *Stress is everywhere, so how can we manage it?* First of all you need to know that you are under stress ... this means you have to be in touch with your body and its reactions to stress. Next, it's important to make a list of your priorities. Work on simple problems first, and then move on to more difficult concerns. Break down those difficult tasks into smaller goals and you will find yourself making great strides in accomplishing your goals.

▶ *Is it true that the most popular techniques for reducing stress are the best ones?* Stress reduction can be different for everyone. Some people may benefit from yoga, others meditation. Some people reduce stress with exercise, while others relax by listening to music. Each of us has different means of dealing with stressors; the key is to discover a program that works for you.

Quick tips for stress reduction

▶ Participate in a cancer support group
▶ Exercise on a regular basis
▶ Make time for yourself. Do something you enjoy like watching a movie, knitting, shooting baskets, or going for a walk
▶ Eat nutritionally healthy foods
▶ Get plenty of sleep and maintain a consistent sleep schedule, or ask your doctor to prescribe a sleep aid
▶ Learn to say "no"
▶ Establish your priorities and stick to them
▶ Learn to establish realistic expectations of yourself
▶ Learn meditation, progressive muscle relaxation, yoga or some other form of stress management
▶ Practice deep breathing
▶ Play with your pet
▶ Read a good book

Jeannie, 60, says, "I went to exercise classes at our local health club (with) no hair and all through chemo. I must have had 15 or 20 women tell me that there is life after breast cancer. They knew I was pretty numb and upset in the beginning, but they were wonderful. They were so much encouragement to me, and the exercise felt good, too, even though some days that was about all I was able to handle physically."

Finding balance: Some common tips for caregivers

▶ *Be open with your loved one.* Tell them your limits with time, financial resources, and your ability to assist with transportation or other tasks.

▶ *Discuss important issues with your loved one, even though the discussions might be uncomfortable.* Discuss finances, insurance coverage, co-payments, and means of accessing funds to care for your loved one's medical needs.

▶ *Discuss options for assisted living, if necessary.* Yes, this might be a difficult subject, but in some cases, you may not be able to provide the type of medical assistance your loved one needs.

▶ *Discuss living wills, issues of "death and dignity," your loved one's desires for medical care, or limitations on medical assistance if the disease is terminal.*

▶ *Investigate community resources so you can access assistance available in your community.*

▶ *Talk with your loved one about things they want to accomplish.* This helps you know what they *really* need and desire, without creating a situation where you feel like you need to do everything.

▶ *Discuss the importance of all members of the family assisting with taking care of the loved one.* If one member is doing all the caretaking, there is an opportunity for resentment and anger to be part of the family dynamics.

▶ *Find ways to balance your own life and responsibilities with your place of employment.* Talk to your employer and discuss possible ways to integrate some extended time away, flexible hours, or perhaps family medical leave.

▶ *Try to maintain some portion of your life in a "normal" fashion.* This may be something as simple as getting up at the same time each day, and going to bed at the same time each night. Normality can include maintaining a consistent nutritious life style, continuing that morning exercise class, or not giving up your monthly book club gathering.

▶ *Make time to renew your own strength.* If you aren't taking care of yourself, it's impossible for you to care for anyone else.

The 'perfect caregiver'

Do you feel you aren't doing all you should be doing, or dealing with the cancer "good enough?" Do you believe that you must give 110 percent to your loved one for fear that you will be seen as a failure?

Perfectionists create self-defeating thoughts and behaviors aimed at achieving unrealistic and excessively high goals. Ultimately this pattern creates poor self-esteem and a feeling of failure because the individual believes they are incapable of achieving anything "worthy" or "enough."

Perfectionism robs us of personal satisfaction and feeling positive about our accomplishments and our future success. Many perfectionists feel intense anxiety about themselves due to the fear of people's criticism, fear of their disapproval, and thoughts of disappointing people who we view as important.

What can you do if you discover you are a perfectionist?

▸ *Set realistic expectations.* You have to make time for yourself, and you can't take care of your survivor 24 hours a day, and still care for yourself.

▸ *Set small goals to assure success.* Make sure you keep things simple!

▸ *Focus on the process not the end point* (the journey, not the destination!)

▸ *Focus on successes.* Acknowledge the positive actions you are doing for your survivor, your loved ones, and for yourself

▸ *Confront the fear* … but allow yourself to be human and make mistakes.

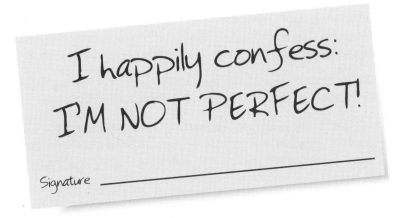

I happily confess:
I'M NOT PERFECT!

Signature _____

Quick relaxation techniques for patients or loved ones

226

There are a wealth of things we can do when we are under stress. Some of the techniques suggested below are time honored, and we have used all of them at various times. Any of these may work for you, especially if you tune into your stress and your need for relaxation. The key is being alert to your need for relaxation! Here are some quick relaxation suggestions:

▶ *Take a five-minute break.* Take a walk, sit or lie down quietly. Perhaps chatting with a support member for a few minutes would also be helpful.

▶ *Take a short nap.* A 15 to 30-minute nap can be as rejuvenating as a night's sleep.

▶ *Spend a few minutes imagining a peaceful, relaxing scene or event in your life.* Recall it in detail, and try to imagine what it felt like utilizing all of your senses. You could also imagine something pleasant that you are looking forward to doing in the near future, or a way in which you reward yourself.

▶ *Massage your forehead, your eyes, your neck muscles, or your back.* Additionally, you might learn some trigger points utilized by certified massage therapists to reduce tension.

▶ *Breathe deeply.* Take a deep breath, let it go deeply into your abdomen. Hold it for the count of five, and then exhale slowly.

▶ *Close your eyes.* Visualize your muscles becoming relaxed and less tense. Try to imagine a white light that is entering the area of pain or tension and evaporating all of the stress.

▶ *Run outside, exercise.* Go outside and yell or scream (obviously, not in a large crowd). Stretch your muscles or do yoga.

▶ *Do something calming like petting a dog or hugging a cat.* Do some knitting, or go outside and shoot some baskets. Perhaps doing a crossword puzzle, or watching a humorous television show will lower your stress level.

Give yourself the precious gift of sleep

Is lost sleep an important issue for caregivers? Ask anyone who has missed a few nights sleep. Sleep is just as essential as food, air and water. Since this is a common concern for many survivors, family, and friends, we offer some suggestions to assist.

If you suffer with insomnia, you may want to consider some of the following suggestions. First of all, never oversleep. Get up at the same time every day even after you have lost sleep. Sleeping late just resets your body clock to a different cycle. Secondly, you must remember to "set your body clock." Light helps restart your body clock to its daytime phase. When you get up, it is essential to get some sunlight into the room, or turn on all the lights. Make sure you walk around to get oxygen to your brain.

Next, make sure you get lots of exercise. Even though you are tired, it is important to keep active during the day, especially after a bad night's sleep. Research indicates that when you sleep less, you should be more active the next day. Try strenuous exercise in late afternoon versus late at night. Don't nap! When you feel sleepy go take a walk or do errands and don't allow yourself to nap. It will only insure you won't sleep tonight! Lastly, set a bedtime schedule. Try to go to bed at the same time each night. If you have lost sleep the night before, go to bed a little later *not earlier* and then move it back to its original time.

For cancer patients, some chemo treatments induce insomnia due to the percentage of steroids. This can affect a patient's sleep patterns significantly. They need to keep track of sleeplessness and report any medical issues regarding medications with their oncologist.

Here are some ideas that researchers suggest for most people:

▶ *Take a warm bath and never a shower before bed.* Long warm baths soothe and unwind tense muscles, leaving you relaxed enough to sleep.

▶ *Try to stretch and relax. Read a boring book or do something, which is a repetitive calming activity.* Do something that puts your mind at rest. Try imagining yourself next to a waterfall. It is much more effective than trying to count sheep!

▸ *Make sure you don't eat immediately before you sleep.* Try to eat at least four hours before you go to sleep.

▸ *Try warm milk at bedtime, which stimulates the serotonin in your body.* Try a piece of whole-wheat bread or other carbohydrates that helps induce sleep. Don't forget the powerful effects of turkey or tuna fish sandwiches ... they really do induce sleep because they are rich in amino acids.

228

▸ *Avoid coffee, colas, tea, chocolate, fermented cheese, cheddar cheese, avocados and red wines.* Research indicates these things keep many people awake at night. Some research suggests it is best to avoid any caffeine or soft drinks, which contain stimulants, after lunchtime and throughout the night.

▸ *Avoid more than 1 or 2 servings of alcohol at dinnertime or during the rest of the night.* Some people believe alcohol will serve as a sedative, but it actually disrupts sleep.

▸ *Don't watch anything disturbing before bed.* Avoid action shows, movies with violence, thrillers, horror movies, intense dramas or anything that will keep your mind working overtime. Some people even suggest not watching the news before bedtime.

▸ *Work out your emotional stressors.* Psychological concerns that are unresolved will play havoc with your ability to have successful sleep. Try to ban worry from the bedroom and do not rehash the events of the day while you are lying in bed.

▸ *Try to avoid drinking liquids 2-3 hours before going to sleep.* Insomnia is often linked to our need to get up and go to the bathroom, which only disrupts your sleep cycle.

▸ *Remember to keep your room around 60-65 degrees and pile on another blanket if you get cold.* Make sure you keep humidity in the room, because dry rooms don't make for good sleep conditions.

▸ *Eliminate noises that keep you awake.* Try using white noise, a fan running, or play relaxing music to block out disruptive noise.

▸ *Set your "body clock" to sleep by keeping the room as dark as possible.* Light in a room tells the body it is time to wake up.

Try these suggestions and have a good night's sleep!

Depression: How to recognize the signs and battle them

Everyone feels "down" or "in the "dumps" at different times in their life. Sadness, loneliness, unhappiness are all a normal part of life. But, when the feelings linger for weeks or months and prevent us from functioning in a healthy or positive manner, it could signal depression.

A common experience among many cancer survivors and caregivers, depression can increase the devastating impact of the cancer diagnosis. Research indicates that depression is the most common mental health concern of Americans, affecting millions of people each year. Some researchers believe that 5 percent of our society is affected by depression at any given time. It is believed that 10-25 percent of Americans will experience major depression at some time in their lives. Statistics also indicate women are twice as likely as males to be affected by depression.

Common signs of depression include:

▸ Depressed mood
▸ Loss of interest in activities
▸ Dissatisfaction with life
▸ Withdrawal from friends, family, and activities
▸ Loss of energy
▸ Irritability
▸ Sadness and crying
▸ Difficulty concentrating or making decisions
▸ Loss of appetite and weight (less commonly increased sleep and weight gain)
▸ Worry and self-critical thoughts
▸ Suicidal thoughts
▸ Substance abuse

The good news is that depression is highly treatable, and the recovery rate is over 85 percent. There are several approaches to treatment, with the most common being "talk therapy." Most commonly a treatment option is suggested by oncologists and cancer centers. Today's facilities are routinely offering therapy as an integral part of a medical model of recovery for cancer patients and

229

family members. Therapy helps people identify the issues that contribute to the depression and teaches coping strategies for minimizing and eliminating depressive symptoms. Therapy also helps pinpoint life concerns that contribute to depression, helping us focus on means for solving or improving the troublesome situations. Therapy helps identify negative or distorted thoughts, which contribute to helplessness and hopelessness. The goal is to regain a sense of control and pleasure in our lives.

Many depressed people also benefit from medication if deemed appropriate. Medication is commonly utilized for moderate or severe depression. Research indicates the most effective treatment for moderate or severe depression is the combination of therapy and medication. But, it is important to realize medication alone will *not* solve the real underlying issues of depression. True recovery can only be accomplished with the integration of therapy to deal with the real issues relating to the depression.

It goes without saying that good nutrition, exercise, sleep, and social involvement help minimize depressive symptoms. Of course, the support and involvement of family and friends are also important assets in recovering from depression. Family and friends can support by encouraging us to express deep feelings and to practice coping skills and problem-solving techniques.

Do I have any signs?

Anxiety can cause much havoc & tear us apart

Just like eating or sleeping, anxiety is a normal part of life. Under the "right" circumstances, anxiety can be beneficial because it motivates us to take action. Faced with an unexpected or unfamiliar challenge, such as cancer, the feeling of anxiety prepares us for the upcoming event. Anxiety heightens our alertness and readies the body for action. Anxiety can also protect us by urging us to take appropriate care of ourself and focus on our immediate needs.

231

Anxiety is something that occurs internally. It is a response or a feeling that something may occur or something is out of our control. Cancer and its diagnosis can create anxiety in many survivors and loved ones. We begin to feel fearful, nervous and incapable of handling the massive stress. Anxiety affects us psychologically, behaviorally and physiologically. Anxiety affects our entire body ... we begin to sweat, our muscles become tense, our heart races, we feel queasy, we have a dry mouth, or we may fear that we will die.

What are some of the most common forms of anxiety disorders?

▶ *Social phobia:* This is the most common anxiety disorder. It involves the fear of embarrassment or humiliation in situations in which you must perform. The fear surrounds the concern that you will say or do something that will cause others to judge you as weak, crazy, or not capable. Some survivors talk about becoming phobic of public activities, fearing people will stare at them because they have no hair. Others talk about being isolated and ignored by friends.

▶ *Specific phobia:* Affecting over 12 percent of all Americans in their lifetime, this type of phobia involves a strong fear or avoidance of one particular type of object or situation. Some of the most common phobias are fear of animals, fear of heights, fear of flying, and fear of blood or needles.

▶ *Generalized anxiety disorder:* This disorder is many times found in survivors and caregivers. It is characterized by anxiety that persists for at least six months. Generally, this occurs when we are concerned about numerous life stresses and experience symptoms of irritability, restlessness, sleeplessness, muscle tension, difficulty concentrating and fatigue.

▶ *Obsessive Compulsive Disorder:* Generally sufferers are reluctant to talk about their symptoms because they impair daily functioning. OCD sufferers might spend hours cleaning, tidying, checking or ordering to the point that these activities interfere with their lives. Some survivors and caregivers take on these behaviors. It seems when you can't control your inner life you try to control your outer life.

232

The most common treatment includes talk therapy with a licensed professional counselor or psychologist. In some cases medication will be added to assist in minimizing symptoms. Some other suggestions for anxiety include:

▶ Do physical exercise

▶ Learn breathing techniques or meditation

▶ Talk to someone in your support network

▶ Use visual distractions (TV, movies, video games)

▶ Use sensory-motor distractions (gardening, crafts, etc)

▶ Find an alternative positive obsession (crossword or jigsaw puzzles)

▶ Practice positive affirmations

Panic attacks affect everyday life dramatically

Affecting over 5 million Americans, panic attacks are characterized by sudden episodes of intense fear or apprehension that may come from "out of the blue." Attacks generally last for a few minutes to an hour. Generally people experience sweating, shortness of breath, racing heart, feeling numb, hot or cold flashes, and fear of going crazy.

Perhaps you might wonder how panic relates to cancer. Survivors and caretakers report that heightened anxiety and fear of impending doom can create panic. These can occur prior to and after diagnosis, during check-ups or other medical procedures.

Studies indicate that 10-22 percent of the adult population will experience a panic attack at some point in their lives. That means that approximately 3 million American will suffer from the effects of this anxiety disorder. These figures don't include the 5 million other Americans who suffer from panic disorder combined with agoraphobia, a disorder in which sufferers are fearful of leaving their homes and experience panic.

Panic disorder usually begins in late teens or in our early 20's and women appear to suffer from panic disorders twice as frequently as men. Some researchers suggest that many males do not report their symptoms, creating the illusion that males suffer less than females.

The American Psychiatric Association defines a panic attack "as an unprovoked surge of fear accompanied by at least four of the following physical and emotional symptoms:"

▸ Shortness of breath or feeling smothered

▸ Dizziness or faintness, trembling or shaking

▸ Sweating or choking

▸ Nausea or abdominal pain or chest discomfort or pain

▸ Numbness or physical sensations

▸ Fear of dying, going crazy or losing control

No one seems to know exactly what causes panic attacks, but most researchers believe there is a biological basis for the disorder. PET scans have shown there is some abnormality in an area of the brain in panic patients. Some panic attacks are triggered by a number of substances or medications. Other people have noticed that caffeine, carbon dioxide, marijuana, and cocaine trigger panic episodes.

But there is help. The first step is to gain an accurate diagnosis from a trained professional counselor who will be able to diagnose the severity of the disorder, and suggest treatment ideas. In some cases medication may be suggested. Generally, the treatment includes psycho-educational training so the sufferer gains a better understanding of the nature of panic, while learning strategies for handling symptoms. Such strategies include relaxation, breathing techniques, and interpreting physical symptoms. Therapists also address other issues related to anxiety to help the sufferer gain more control of their life.

▸ Remember that these are feelings and symptoms, but they are not dangerous or harmful

▸ Breathe in and count to 6; breathe out and count to 6

▸ Learn breathing techniques, and relaxation skills

▸ Try not to fight the feelings. Relax and breathe deeply and the panic symptoms will pass

▸ Tell yourself something calming such as "This will pass" or "I can stay calm."

▸ Try to focus on something that will take your mind off the symptoms. Try counting backwards from 100 by 3's, sing a song in your head, or do some multiplication in your mind.

▸ Notice that when you stop thinking about being afraid or that you might die, the frightening thoughts and anxiety fade.

Anger takes its toll on the body, mind and soul

Feeling angry now and then is a normal response, especially when the anger is due to a specific event, such as cancer, or interpersonal situations. But for some people, anger and hostility are long-term habits or personality traits.

What happens to your body when you get angry? Anger triggers physical responses which include: a racing heart, an increase in blood pressure, muscle tension, stomach ailments, back pain and dilation of the arteries. Your body starts to prepare for the "fight or flight syndrome." The body also releases stress chemicals and over time, which can contribute to clogged arteries. Anger can damage your heart muscle, produce heart attacks and increase your chance for cancer.

Here are a few healthy suggestions for dealing with anger:

▸ Talk about difficult situations with a trusted friend or family member

▸ Slow down. Think before you act out of habit or impulse.

▸ Learn to assess and read your body so you know when anger is building inside you. Learn where you hold anger (back pain, stomach ailments, migraines, etc.)

▸ Know your triggers and try to avoid them

▸ Look for humor in the situation

▸ Exercise on a regular basis

▸ Talk yourself down when you feel anger coming on

▸ When you feel anger coming on, take 3-5 deep breaths

▸ Take a time out, count to 10, or take a walk

▸ Learn some new ways to communicate assertively vs. aggressively

▸ Practice relaxation techniques

▸ Practice meditation or visualization

▸ Talk to a licensed professional who can assess anger concerns and teach anger management techniques

The painful blame game: No one will ever win

Some secrets can be devastating. Many of our survivors secretly talked about feeling they were "responsible" for bringing cancer to themselves. Others said that family members insisted that "I should have done more ... fought harder in the early stages." These messages are physically, emotionally and spiritually battering to everyone.

There is no blame or guilt with cancer ... no one asks for cancer to invade their body. It isn't something anyone wants.

But honestly, doesn't it cross our mind when someone who smokes gets lung cancer? "Well, if they hadn't smoked, they wouldn't have gotten cancer." Not all smokers get lung cancer. Non-smokers also get it. Sometimes there's no reason at all for lung cancer.

And what about someone who drank alcohol heavily for a long time and they get cancer of the liver? Do we blame them for causing their cancer? Not all alcoholics get cancer of the liver. Non-alcoholics also get it. Sometimes there's no reason at all for cancer of the liver.

And what about the person who doesn't eat a healthy diet and gets colon cancer? Do we point an accusing finger at those individuals, chastising them for not getting enough fiber? Not all people with bad diets get colon cancer. Health food junkies also get it. Sometimes there's no reason at all for colon cancer.

And what about the sun worshipper who gets skin cancer? Do we target them for causing their own condition? Not all people who are over-exposed to the sun get skin cancer. People who stay out of the sun also get skin cancer. Sometimes there's no reason at all for skin cancer.

Blame. We often need to blame something or someone for cancer because we're so angry at the diagnosis. People are real. We can see their bad habits or behaviors. We can't see the cancer cells that have mysteriously mutated and spread their deadly trail silently in the body.

Imagine the cancer patient who looks in the mirror every day, wondering, agonizing over what they did wrong, what one mistake did they make, what did they forget to do or check.

This isn't the time for blame or self-doubt. This is the time to battle the *real* enemy, cancer. Who cares how it may have started. We should only care how we're going to destroy it before it destroys us.

Get over it!?

236

What's holding me back?

What has made me angry while confronting cancer? _____

_____

Have I blamed myself or my loved one for this cancer? Why? _____

_____

_____

_____

How can I get past blame? How can I focus on the healing process?

_____

_____

Are there old emotional wounds that have not healed? How can I

turn that around and start anew? _____

_____

_____

_____

How can I allow myself to forgive those who have hurt me?

_____

_____

_____

Changing habits may be part of recovery

Do you remember the movie "Ground Hog Day"? In this comedy, Bill Murray keeps waking up to the same day over and over again until he learns to change his attitude and the way he is addressing people in his life. This is an excellent analogy for those who continue doing the same thing over and over and expecting different results. "If you do what you did, you will always get what you got!"

The thought of making personal changes excites many people, but for most, the thought of change is very fearful. When a suggestion is made that we might need to change our behavior or thinking pattern, most people are filled with fear. Change is a scary thing for most people because of the unpredictability of the results. On the other hand, doing something the same way seems to insure failure!

The diagnosis of cancer mandates change. Cancer turns our lives upside down and only we can decide if we will come up on top, or allow the adversity to destroy our life. With this in mind, here are some suggestions for those people who have a difficult time setting goals and making changes:

▸ *First of all, examine the situation.* You must know the full extent of the problem or concern before you can create a change.

▸ *Try to identify the source of the problem.* Does the change involve a person, place, or event, or something in your control? Are you trying to change something that is out of your control? If it is out of your control (like the diagnosis of cancer), then the thing you *can* change is the way you react to the cancer.

▸ *Try to understand the dynamics of the problem.* Investigate what you typically do to create the same harmful behaviors. It is essential to discover your part in the problem and be aware of the usual and consistent pitfalls that create failures.

▸ *Look for alternatives.* Are there other options or ways you can change your behavior that you have not tried? Can you brainstorm some other ways to think about the problem? Can you try another approach and change your behavior in this situation?

▶ *Rehearse new behaviors.* Practice makes perfect. Remember, research indicates it takes 21 days to create change. Try reinforcing these with some positive affirmations!

▶ *Be specific about your goal and know exactly what you want to happen.* Visualize your cancer being eliminated with your new thoughts.

238 ▶ *Know why you are making the change.* It is essential that you know the importance of your goal, especially if you are tempted to slip or quit because you don't see immediate results.

▶ *Is this change relevant to your life?* Is it important to you? Change can only occur when you are dedicated to bringing about a new way of behaving or looking at the problem.

"Change has a considerable psychological impact on the human mind. To the fearful it is threatening because it means that things may get worse. To the hopeful it is encouraging because things may get better. To the confident it is inspiring because the challenge exists to make things better." King Whitney Jr.

Caring for me

Self-care for survivors, caregivers, loved ones and friends

How and where can I find the time I need to be alone to "re-group"

or "re-energize"? _____

_____

How can I make sure I'm eating nutritiously and at regular intervals?

_____

_____

How and where can I find the time to give myself a break and visit

with friends? _____

_____

How do I maintain a support network of family and friends who can

give me the emotional outlet I need? _____

_____

_____

How do I now define "quality time" with loved ones and friends?

How am I going to make that time? _____

_____

_____

Just one of many
Thoughts about facing fear

240

"Perfect love casteth out fear"

When I become fearful, I think about why I am afraid. I ask what is the worst thing that can happen. Then I focus on verses in the Bible like "What time I am afraid I will trust in thee." I will count on God's grace to get me through whatever it is that I have to face. Focusing on God's love for me and on the fact that HE will never leave me or forsake me helps calm my fears.

M

It has taken me a long time to see that there are differences between the fear of dying and the sadness about dying. My fear is not dying. My fear is about the process of dying and the pain involved. Perhaps I've heard too many horror stories of uncontrollable pain, though, I have seen three deaths that were peaceful, and without it.

When I realized that my feelings of actually dying were really those of sadness, I began to feel selfish in some ways. I've had a very blessed life – not without hard times – but with lots of learning and love. My sadness is for things I haven't experienced, like seeing my grandchildren grow up, having them know me. Yet, I have seen them. Gradually, I am learning to let go of sadness and truly know that being alive today can never be taken away and is the real source of joy. I will be alive to them through my family and children.

241

B

"Overcome fear, behold wonder"
I behold the wonder of life as I see my new grandson. Life will continue through him even if my own life stops. I also wonder at my own grandparents. I continued their work and joy. I have thought of them even more than my own parents. I hope that I can continue the wonder of the continuity of family — the sister's nose, great-grandfather's face shape, my mother's eyes. All coming together in this wondrous new life. What is there to fear? I will be forever.

J

If we believe in God, He gives us daily grace to live by and He promises dying grace when we have need of it. Therefore we must believe His word when he says, "Fear not."

T

"It is not death that men should fear, but he should fear never beginning to live." Marcus Aelius Aurelius, (121-180 AD) Roman Emperor, Philosopher

242

Being faced with cancer or other life-threatening illnesses seems to have both positive and negative sides. I think fear is the first and deepest emotion I have felt. Once that eases a bit, I can look at my life and realize how lucky I have been. I do a life review, even though I am not quite middle-aged yet. I am happy with my life and realize this is a very good life, which some people never get.

Death comes to all of us as did birth. I start from God and return to Him. I will always hold some fear because it is unknown, but being happy with life is a good start.

Robin

Fear is something I haven't experienced since the first couple of months after my initial diagnosis of cancer. When I was originally diagnosed, I learned what real fear felt like. I was consumed with thoughts of not only what I wouldn't be able to do for myself, but more for what I might not be able to do for others, particularly my family. Every thought, every word, every action brought with it a set of circumstances that fear could rule over. It was a terrible downward spiral without end.

I want to be there for my children, for all the moments of their lives when they need their mother. From laundry to driving, dating, college, marriage and raising their own children. I feel strongly that guidance through all these issues is essential, from both parents, to successfully blossom into strong independent productive adults.

I want to be there for my husband, to keep him warm at night, to tell him I love him, to share a lifetime of memories.

I want to be there for parents, who were always supporting me, every step of the way. They have health issues and are needing someone to be there for them, and I hope I can always be.

I want to be there for my brother, who I am very close to. We have always discussed all the major issues of our lives.

Fear to me is cancer stopping me from being there for those who need me; so, I refuse to let fear enter my life any more. I keep busy taking care of the people in my life who have always taken care of me, and don't allow time for fear to enter my life any more.

D

243

The power of prayer

No matter the religious affiliation or beliefs or even absence of such, most people turn to prayer to help them through a difficult situation. In fact, prayer and faith were listed as the most utilized coping skill sited by survivors and loved ones in our surveys.

It's important to understand that you do not need to share the same beliefs to pray with someone. Prayer is about having a spiritual opening to something greater ... it isn't necessarily about religion. Prayer is personal, a reflection of our life experiences, a soul enriched call for strength, peace, miracles, acceptance, answers. Sitting with someone or a group in silence as each reaches deep within for the appropriate words can be comforting. The sense of having someone close by — physically and spiritually — gives us the courage to relax and focus on what we spiritually need to get through tough times. Your inner voice will be clearer and more meaningful.

And because we're human, frustrated or afraid, we can have "angry" prayers, too, which can be a natural part of the grieving process, including a questioning of and anger toward God or other higher power. Some people subscribe to the belief that God never gives us more than we can handle.

Here is what some of our survivors and loved ones had to say about prayer and faith.

▶ The Bible and God's promise of a paradise. *Betty, 74, NA*

▶ God and His healing touch. Philippians 4:13: "I can do all things through Christ who strengthened me." *Rosalie, 80, breast*

▶ I understand sometimes you have to have your time alone with God. *Bambi, 47, mother and sister, breast*

▶ My faith in God. I knew that God knew I could handle it with His help. He wouldn't have given it to me if there's wasn't some good that would come out of it. *Martha, 51, breast*

▶ We will put this in God's hands and pray. If God wills it, we will get well and go on with our life. *Alveretta, 85, ovarian*

▶ Have patience. Pray to God and have a lot of faith. *Patricia, 73, breast*

▶ Yes, she told me she was not afraid to die and about her belief in the power of prayer and joining her loved ones who had already passed away. *Tracy, 47, mother, lung*

▶ Acceptance of God's will, whatever that was. *Bette, 57, husband, melanoma*

▶ (Friend was helped by her) knowledge of heaven and assurance she will be going there. Friends, family, her faith, belief in Jesus, encouragement from people, church family and Sunday school class. *Kathleen, 49, friend, breast*

▶ Ask if they have a workable faith in God. *John, 81, prostate and colon*

▶ Read all the material and be prepared. Talk about it to friends. Keep an open mind but most of all trust in God. He'll see you through this. *V, 64, breast*

▶ Pray. It works. *Maria, 61, breast*

▶ We decided to take things one day at a time and that we'd never give up hope. She had tremendous faith. *Hiles, 69, wife, uterine*

▶ He had the faith needed, we both did. Left it in God's hands. *L, 66, husband, prostrate*

My prayers

✏ _____

✏ _____

✏ _____

✏ _____

✏ _____

✏ _____

Meditation calms body and soul

246

Meditation is simply a means of quieting down your thoughts. It is a method for slowing down a racing mind to gain awareness, insight, and a connection with your inner spiritual self. The purpose or intention is to direct your concentration on healing and fill you with peace and tranquility. For thousands of years, those who practice mediation on a regular basis, have found the practice lowers stress levels, decreases impulsive actions, minimizes burnout, and helps to heal a body that is affected by trauma, disease, or illnesses such as cancer. Additionally, recent studies show that meditation lowers our blood pressure and heart rate, assists with enhancing our concentration, lowers anxiety, fear and worry.

Meditation helps survivors and loved ones attain an understanding of their inner feelings, and reduces feelings of hopelessness and helplessness. Meditation is also a very useful form of stress reduction which helps to eliminate negative thoughts.

You don't have to be a Maharishi or a yogi to perform meditation. All you need is a quiet spot and the desire to quiet your mind. Find a comfortable sitting position (sitting straight backed or assisted by a wall). Allow your mind to be calm. Breathe in and out counting each inhale to 6 or 8. Focus on your breathing and allow your mind to open. Some who meditate focus on bringing white healing light into the body; or visualize sitting on a beach, by a babbling brook, or on a mountain top. Others recite words such as "calm" or "peace" over and over. *You choose!* The key is slowing the mind and allowing your body the opportunity to heal itself.

Breast cancer survivor Lorraine explains her experience:

I have for a long time believed strongly in the mind/body connection in relationship to physical and emotional health. Actually putting it to use during diagnosis, chemo, surgery, radiation and post-treatment emotional difficulties had results almost too big to put in words. I used mostly visualization during treatment, and feel it had the most profound results in treating my cancer. When I was diagnosed, I had three tumors in my breast and in a lymph node (which was described as being the size of a billiard ball). I had eight chemo treatments, followed by surgery. Thirteen lymph nodes were removed, with no sign of cancer. There were no active cancer cells in the affected node! I also had an amazing number of people praying for me. I so strongly believe in the power of prayer and feel this is what led to my outcome.

The power of touch

It seems so simple, but often the simple parts of life are ignored. One of these necessities is the powerful essence of the human touch.

▶ Holding hands

▶ Hugs

▶ A gentle hand on the shoulder

▶ Holding a loved one non-sexually in bed (spooning)

▶ Rubbing gently on the back

▶ Massaging temples of the head

▶ Kiss on the cheek

Some survivors have indulged in massage therapy, though that is something that first should be approved by your doctor. A therapist who specializes in working with cancer patients is recommended.

"*Rub their feet, neck, back or whatever they say would make them feel better.*"
Diane, 47, breast

Lorraine had been seeing a "wonderful" massage therapist until her life was disrupted with the diagnosis of cancer. She took a break and went back only with her physician's approval after completing her cancer treatment.

She appreciates the way her massage therapist helped her relax and escape a "million miles away" from reality through a simple back rub or massaging of her feet. Her therapist also gave her some relaxation techniques that have been a vital part of her healing process. The mere sensation of touch has been beneficial and made her feel more connected to the world that continued to evolve around her as she battled cancer.

"*My husband never hovered over me, but would from time to time put his arms around me and ask how things were going.*" Carolyn, 70, colon

'I'm meeting her needs, not mine': noble, not real

248   Reading through the surveys, we stopped at one written by a loved one. The author wrote, "I'm meeting her needs, not mine." It was heartfelt, compassionate and noble, but perhaps not realistic in the long run.

It may sound selfish, but if we do not meet our own physical and emotional needs first, we can't help anyone else. It's like they tell you on an airplane: In case of an emergency, put on **your** oxygen mask first and then take care of your children or those who need assistance around you. If you aren't okay, then you can't help anyone around you. If you're strong and focused, you can help many more people.

The same is true for those who care for cancer patients or anyone facing a health emergency. It's easy to forget to eat or sleep when you're so focused on someone else. We know the adrenaline will carry us through a temporary crisis. It has so far.

Well, sooner or later, that miraculous well of energy will evaporate. You're not going to be able to help anyone if you've collapsed from exhaustion. Yes, we are amazingly resilient creatures, but we're only human.

What do I need?

✏ _____

✏ _____

✏ _____

✏ _____

✏ _____

Affirmations can create serenity

Affirmations can be a powerful ally to imprint positive statements into your subconscious. Affirmations are personal, positive and present tense statements, which are written in an effort to alter negative thoughts or patterns.

249

Affirmations should be:

▶ *Stated in the present tense, which means in the "now"* ("I accept … I feel … I give")

▶ *Affirmations should be positive* ("I am … I will … I deserve …")

▶ *Affirmations should be repeated at least 10 times a day for a minimum of 21 days.* Proven in numerous studies, this methodology is the practice of meditation guru Ruth Fishel.

▶ *You should feel good about what you are saying to yourself* ("I am happily whole and healthy, I accept myself completely, I can bring recovery to my body")

▶ *You begin to act and feel as if your statements are true and realistic*

▶ *Use positive action words.* "I easily … I quickly … I show…"

▶ *Visualize your own success.* Feel the emotion that goes with the success.

▶ *Be realistic about your affirmation statement.*

▶ *Adhere to the old Alcoholics Anonymous statement, "Fake it until you make it."* Affirmations may seem uncomfortable, or you might have negative self-talk, but keep going like you believe it, and it will meet with success! Trust us…It will become part of your belief system.

Affirmations can be used:

▶ *Silently while meditating or relaxing*

▶ *On tape.* You can make your own tape of affirmations or purchase a pre-produced affirmation tape

▶ *Written.* This is the most powerful method and remember to do them ten times a day for at least 21 days!

▶ *Recited aloud.* You can do this while you take a walk, in the car, or while exercising. And it is okay to talk to yourself. People won't think you are crazy!

Affirmations

250

What statements will help me?

Write three affirmations for yourself. Make sure they are positive, in the present tense, personal and specific of what you want to happen.

1. _____

_____

_____

2. _____

_____

_____

3. _____

_____

_____

"Affirmations are like prescriptions for certain aspects of yourself you want to change."
Jerry Frankhauser

Getting it down on paper

Putting our thoughts down on paper during difficult times is one of the greatest gifts we can give to ourselves and others. Many individuals keep journals to chart their path and progress through cancer. Journals often become a confidante to absorb a multitude of words and emotions, both good and bad.

251

No matter the writing instrument or surface, keep in mind the following:

▸ It can be anything from an elegant leather journal to scraps of paper, just write it

▸ It doesn't matter what you write, just write it

▸ Forget every grammar rule your high school English teacher taught you, just write it

▸ Scribble your thoughts and throw them away later if you want, just write it

▸ Keep a mini shredder nearby for when you're really mad

Now you ask, what do you do with your journal(s) or other items written in anger earlier? Loved ones need to know that we all have feelings, and sometimes those feelings are not pleasant to hear. A journal is a private means to sort our feelings, and it should be kept that way … If by chance someone does find a journal, we think it would be important to remember that these are "just feelings" and the importance of the journal is to help someone sort out those feelings and that a personal journal was never meant for someone else to read.

"Every time I had a chemo treatment, I would picture the drugs going into my body and finding and destroying any cancer cell that was out there. I also kept a diary of my battle with cancer. I look back on it now and am so proud that I was able to accomplish all of this and am still around to enjoy life!" Melinda, 46, breast

Pet therapy may be what the doc ordered

252

Can pets really have an effect on our physical and mental health? The answer is a strong resounding … YES! In fact, research shows that pets lower the owner's depression level, raise life expectancy, and increase our physical health.

However, it is important to note that some cancer patients have to find temporary or permanent arrangements for a pet due to their current medical status with immune system impairments, etc. This can be a tremendous adjustment to say the least, so be prepared for this possibility. This could affect the entire family, so be sure and sit down and talk about the options together because pets are often considered a member of the family.

A recent study investigated a group of patients who owned an animal, versus those who did not own a pet. The research findings indicated that pet owners had lower blood pressure compared to those patients who did not own a pet. In fact, another study discovered the act of talking to a pet can actually decrease blood pressure.

What are some of the other benefits of having a pet?

▸ In a study of more than 1,000 Medicare patients, dog owners in the study had 21 percent fewer physician contacts than non-dog owners.

▸ Pets give unconditional love and support; undivided loyalty and devotion; total acceptance and nurturing. They make us feel appreciated and seem to increase our sense of self-esteem and worth.

▸ Pets provide a sense of security and protection.

▸ Pets are wonderful companions and eliminate our feelings of loneliness and isolation.

▸ Pets have been shown to be a help with stress and its symptoms.

▸ Pets ease loss. Survivors with pets are less likely to experience deterioration in health following stressful events.

▸ Pets encourage survivors to become more active.

▸ Pets encourage our survivors to take better care of themselves because they have something to love and nurture.

Girls/boys night in

Need a break? Need a party? Need to laugh? Need to just be around your friends? Need to forget reality for awhile?

Consider having a girls or boys night in. The survivor may not have the energy to go out but may welcome the opportunity to see familiar faces, laugh and just have fun.

▶ Order in pizza

▶ Have someone make and bring the survivor's favorite food

▶ Have a cook out

▶ Decorate hats, caps, scarves or tur-
bans with fun designs and bright
colors for the survivor to wear

▶ Watch DVD's or videos

▶ Watch old home movies

▶ Go through old photo albums or
scrapbooks

▶ Play board games

▶ Play cards

▶ Just talk

It doesn't have to be a night out or in. It can any time of the day or week or year or in any place. It can be a day of shopping or at a sport-ing event. It can be friends forming a team to run or walk in honor of the survivor when the survivor can't be there in person. It's just all about being together for the survivor and each other.

> "My friends visited one weekend. We sat up, laughed and talked. Even though I fell asleep early, I was comforted by knowing they were with me." Diane, 47, breast

▶ We had the "girls" get together for some laughs. *Melinda, 46, breast*

▶ Get away for a while, movie, dinner, salon! *Tracy, 33, cervical*

▶ We party and joke about it and prayed. My friends are super and very caring. *V, 64, breast*

▶ They listened. Got together and purchased a day at the spa. They participate in the Race for the Cure each year with me. *Karen, 33, breast*

Humor is a great healer

254

The movie "Patch Adams" clearly addressed the importance of utilizing humor, a vital part of the healing process for those suffering with life-threatening diseases. Most currently, groups like Rx Laughter have been organized to assist chronically ill children and teens through the use of funny television shows and movies during their treatment process. Laughter enhances their immune functions, speeds up their rate of healing, and tends to minimize the pain experienced during difficult procedures.

Hundreds of studies have examined the correlation between laughter, humor and the healing capacity of the activity. Our survivors agree with these studies and many reported the importance of watching funny movies, laughing at cartoons, hearing some good jokes, and having a daily dose of laughter.

It is essential for our physical and mental health to place a little laughter and humor into the lives of survivors, family, friends and other loved ones. We encourage you to do a few of these silly things and have a few laughs …

▸ At lunchtime, sit in your parked car wearing sunglasses and point a hair dryer at passing cars. See if they slow down.

▸ Every time someone asks you to do something, ask them if they want fries with that.

▸ As often as possible, skip rather than walk.

▸ Specify that your drive-through order is "to go."

▸ Call the psychic hotline and say nothing.

▸ Go to your bank's ATM machine. Wait until there's a crowd around you, and when the money comes out of the ATM machine scream, "I won, I won!"

▸ Tell your best friend, "It's not the voices in my head that bother me. It's the voices in your head that do."

▸ Tell your children over dinner, "Due to the economy, we are going to have to let one of you go."

▸ When you leave the zoo, start running towards the parking lot yelling, "Run for your lives, they're loose!"

▸ Learn a new joke every day and make your loved ones listen to it. If they don't laugh, tell them the joke again and again until they break into laughter.

So have a little fun and smile … it's a small step towards a happy outlook, and a positive attitude.

There are times...

I (Joy Miller) have come to realize that there are just certain times in our lives when we want to "run away." I realize that the term "running away" has different connotations for each other us. For me, I just want to run away and live on a puppy ranch where I can spend the entire day rejoicing in puppies' kisses and licks. I'll run through the fields with all types of little pups and just laugh, giggle and relax. I do realize that this might not be everyone's fantasy plan for running away ... but it is surely my dream when things get overwhelming and life seems to run into itself.

As a therapist, I tell my clients to breath ... live in the moment ... stay focused on what really matters in your life. I advise my clients to stay out of their own self-destructive thoughts and use calming relaxation techniques. I've even suggested that clients make personalized affirmation tapes to remind them of their purpose and goals in life.

But, sometimes all the therapeutic techniques in the world just don't seem to be "just the right solution." The following contract is my new plan for life. I've decided that I must take some radical action, or I may forget to live life with the passion in which it was intended. So here goes...

I, _____, hereby officially tender my resignation as an adult. I have decided I would like to accept the responsibilities of an 8 year old again. I want to go to McDonald's and think that it's a four star. I want to sail sticks across a fresh mud puddle and make ripples with rocks. I want to think M&Ms are better than money because you can eat them. I want to lie under a big oak tree and run a lemonade stand with my friends on a hot summer's day. I want to return to a time when life was simple. When all you knew were colors, multiplication tables, and nursery rhymes, but that didn't bother you, because you didn't know what you didn't know and you didn't care. All you knew was to be happy because you were blissfully unaware of all the things that should make you worried or upset. I want to think the world

"Laughter gives us distance. It allows us to step back from an event, deal with it and then move on." Bob Newhart

is fair. That everyone is honest and good. I want to believe that anything is possible. I want to be oblivious to the complexities of life and be over excited by the little things again. I want to live simple again. I don't want my day to consist of computer crashes, mountains of paperwork, depressing news, how to survive more days in the month than there is money in the bank, doctor bills,

> "We cannot really love anybody with whom we never laugh."
> Agnes Repplier

gossip, illness, and loss of loved ones. I want to believe in the power of smiles, hugs, a kind word, truth, justice, peace, dreams, the imagination, mankind, and making angels in the snow. So.... here's my checkbook and my car keys, my credit card bills and my 401K statements. I am officially resigning from adulthood. And if you want to discuss this further, you'll have to catch me first. (Author unknown)

So take some time for yourself and your inner child!

A funny thing happened

A sense of humor was just the medicine Noor needed when she battled breast cancer. She says the laughter took the pain away, even if it was only a temporary reprieve. At least she was not thinking about the disease, and that was quite an enjoyable break.

She explains that while caring for her parents, both of whom had cancer and passed away, she grew personally stronger, and that reinforced her when she faced cancer herself. She describes herself as a very positive person surrounded by a jovial family. That innate humor was already there, and while they didn't ignore her needs, they rarely talked about the cancer and focused instead on life and laughter.

And it paid off.

Though cancer was not a pleasant experience, Mary says she wouldn't give up the life experiences the disease gave her, how it taught her to look at life and the world much differently. One of the greatest healing lessons was and continues to be laughter.

She recalls going out with her wig, but later realized it was gone. It was dark outside as she searched unsuccessfully for the hair piece, which wasn't exactly cheap. The next day, she discovered it on the street near her house. Upon retrieving it, it was immediately evident that a dog had, uh, relieved himself on it.

Nevertheless, Mary gave it a thorough washing as her cat hissed at it. It came through smelling all fresh and clean again, and she wore it when necessary.

And what became of this wig?

She later gave it to another cancer patient.

"And I hope I never see it again," she laughs.

▶ "My two children always knew and felt that their mom could handle about anything. When I lost all of my hair and wore a bandanna, they jokingly said, 'Mom, you look cool. You should get your nose pierced.' " *Vicki, 53, breast*

▶ "Communication and humor (got me through). I loved — not now — 'I'm having a no-hair day.' " *A survivor*

▶ Always keep your sense of humor, even if it is in poor taste. You have to vent somehow and laughter beats crying any time. *Susan, 49, best friend, lymphoma*

▶ Try to keep humor throughout a very difficult ordeal. My sister lost her hair during her treatment, so at Halloween, I went trick or treating with my other sister and a good friend to my sister's house. We wore bald caps. She thought it was great! Some people may not agree, but you know your family/friends better than anyone, so you will know how to help them cope. *Sandi, 51, sister, ovarian*

▶ One sorority sister sent me jokes daily by e-mail. Up to that point, I did not use the computer regularly. *Jeannie, 60, breast*

▶ I asked them to keep it light. They did. Sending funny cards, ridiculous gifts. They stayed in close contact. *Karen, 62, breast*

▶ My best friend supplied humor. We have always been able to laugh together, no matter what. *Rita, 58, breast*

▶ I laughed at myself a lot. This helped me as well as others around me. *Mary, 52, breast*

▶ Be there! Give to them all that was given to you. Listen and be supportive and laugh (at the right times). *Judy, 56, breast*

Consider these simple, yet effective, venues for laughter:

▶ Movies, cartoons, comedy shows, comedians

▶ Old radio shows

▶ Humor, comic, joke and cartoon books

▶ Sunday funny pages

▶ Watching old family movies

▶ Subscribe to online joke a day

'Waiting for the other shoe to drop'

258

Many of our survivors spoke of the fear that their cancer would return. They try to " go on" with life, but secretly they tell us they always live with some fear that the cancer will once again invade their body. Never fully able to enjoy life to the fullest, fear becomes a constant companion.

Here are some suggestions for survivors, loved ones and friends:

▸ *Live for the moment.* Capture the moment, seize the day, and let your heart reach out and feel the joy in this one moment.

▸ *Focus on today and celebrate each and every day.* Start a gratitude journal and keep track of all the celebrations, times of pleasure, and moments with those you love

▸ *Look to the future and continue to plan for longevity and health.* Affirm you will have good health and continue to plan activities with loved ones.

▸ *Say "I love you."* Remember the importance of capturing each day by making sure that you tell those you love just how much they mean to you.

Diane understands the true meaning of surviving cancer:

"Life after surviving cancer is truly a blessing. You view everything differently. I started to think in terms of shorter increments versus looking at doing things next month or five years from now, whether it would be telling someone I love them, trying to help someone in need, or accomplishing a goal."

"As a survivor, you must remember when you hear of a friend's cancer diagnosis that it's NOT YOU. This may sound selfish, but it helps you to cope and keep a healthy perspective."
A survivor

When treatment is over: What then?

No matter the type of cancer or treatment, all survivors want to hear the following magical words:

"The cancer appears to be gone. You're in remission. Your treatments are over."

Unfortunately, not everyone gets that pronouncement, though many do and that's glorious news for survivors and their loved ones. Yet, moving on offers challenges of its own, including emotional withdrawal symptoms as your body realigns itself at the same time.

Believe it or not, the transition from treatment to freedom involves the elimination of certain routines that have lasted from months to several years. The security of the treatment process is suddenly gone. Your oncology team has been like a surrogate family in many cases, and there can be grief in that separation, though it may be masked by the joy of absorbing good news.

Survivors have to redefine a "normal" life. **What is that? Is it what life was like before they were diagnosed with cancer?** No. Life will never be the same, and that's an adjustment for the survivor, a shift that has a ripple effect on loved ones and friends, results that can be just as powerful as the cancer itself initiated.

Admit it. Whether it's cancer or something else that requires a new regiment in your life, you tend to adopt an "auto pilot" response. With cancer, it's been treatments or therapy or doctor visits on a regular schedule. Suddenly that "commitment" is gone, and you have the incredible opportunity to take control of your life again.

It sounds easy, but is not as magical as it sounds. For months or years, you've been wearing blinders like a horse in a race, focusing only on winning the race against cancer. Many survivors experience a delayed reaction in adjusting to a cancer-free life, though the disease is often in the back of their minds for a very long time. Some will wonder, *"I should be happy, but I'm not. Why?"*

This requires developing a coping strategy that will help ease that transition from cancer survivor to an ordinary person again.

Maybe it's as simple as grasping how many hours a day or week had been exerted in medical procedures and recovery. Look closely where are all your energies had been focused for so long.

▸ *What will I do with that time now?*

▸ *How many regiments are now over?*

▸ *How many aspects of my life were controlled by the cancer?*

▸ *What will become the new "routines" in my life?*

At the same time, returning to a "normal" life probably means returning to regular household or family chores and a certain role within the family unit.

▸ *How will I take on new or assume old responsibilities?*

▸ *How will I adjust to being "just" a member of the family again?*

At the same time, relationships on all levels will have evolved over time.

▸ *How will I get by without my "chemo pals," upon whom I've become so dependent?*

▸ *How do I maintain those relationships, these individuals who validated what I experienced?*

▸ *What do those relationships mean to me as I've "moved on"?*

▸ *What do I need from all my relationships, family, friends, etc.?*

▸ *Who has and will continue to hold me back if I allow them to?*

▸ *Who will take me where I need to go with my life?*

▸ *How will I find, cultivate and enhance those types of relationships, currently existing or not?*

Cancer has forever changed your view of the world and how your loved ones see that same world. You've all experienced something terribly frightening, and battled the emotional and physical toll that robs survivor, caregiver, family and friends of crucial time.

That is the hidden "gift" of cancer, how it can open the eyes and spirit to the meaning of life and how precious it is. Everyone had to make major changes to fight the survivor's cancer. And now everyone must adopt a new and more meaningful strategy to seize and celebrate that priceless gift.

It need not be complex or threatening.

It can be as simple as saying, "I love you" and meaning it.

Looking back

"Life consists not in holding good cards but in playing those you hold well." Josh Billings

Learning from the past

Our caregivers, family and friends looked at some of their initial reactions to the diagnosis of cancer, and had some thoughts about that time period. Some look back with regret, others feel they did all they could for their loved one. This intimate look into the hearts of our caretakers, family and friends is quite revealing and emotional. Hopefully, this list will be a valuable tool in understanding what our caretakers and friends *wish* they could have done differently, with the wisdom they *now* hold.

▶ I would change nothing
▶ I wish I supported my survivor more even after treatment was finished
▶ I wish I had talked more about death and heaven
▶ I wish I had prayed with my survivor
▶ I wish I asked more questions
▶ I wish I had talked about the illness more
▶ I wish I had taken more time off of work
▶ I wish I had spent more quality time with the my loved one
▶ I wish I had not accepted patient's impending death so easily
▶ I wish I had encouraged patient more to share feelings
▶ I wish I had shared my tears and emotions with my loved one
▶ I wish I had talked more about the survivor's fears / concerns
▶ I wish I had been a better friend
▶ I wish I had not let patient become so dependent on me
▶ I wish I took care of myself better
▶ I wish I had encouraged a more aggressive treatment (lumpectomy vs. mastectomy)
▶ I wish I had been more insistent on a healthier lifestyle for the patient
▶ I wish I had learned more about financial information
▶ I wish I had said "I love you" more
▶ I wish I had been there when patient died
▶ I wish I had encouraged getting a second opinion
▶ I wish I had been more physically affectionate

▸ I wish I had realized the seriousness of the situation
▸ I wish I had listened more
▸ I wish I had researched a better institution/hospital
▸ I wish I had been more open and honest with the survivor
▸ I wish I had kissed patient goodbye when they died
▸ I wish I had moved closer to survivor's hometown
▸ I wish I had accepted others' help
▸ I wish I had helped more
▸ I wish I had quieted the room so we could hear patient's last word
▸ I wish I had been more patient
▸ I wish I had taken them out of hospice care and placed in hospital
▸ I wish I had taken time off school to be with survivor in hospital

263

Top responses

🖉 I would change nothing
🖉 I wish I had spent more quality time with the survivor
🖉 I wish I had shared my tears and emotions with the survivor
🖉 I wish I had said "I love you more"
🖉 I wish I had prayed with the survivor

Loved ones say...

What do you wish you would have said or done differently?

▸ I brought a bunch of books to my mom and told her to look them over and pick one. She read them ALL and was obsessed with telling my dad everything she had learned. He didn't want to hear it! *Laura, 44, father, prostate*

▸ I wish I had known the emotional scars that remain after treatment, the uncertainty of recurrences. *Doug, 57, wife, breast*

▸ I wish I would have argued for the mastectomy instead of the lumpectomy the first time. *John, 55, wife, breast*

▸ I wish we could have talked about his feelings, hopes and achievements. *Julie, 51, father, lung*

▸ Maybe been more insistent, tougher with him to do healthful living for himself. *Judith, 70, husband, colon*

▸ Been better able to be there emotionally. *Bette, 57, husband, melanoma*

▸ I would have talked with her about life and death and eternity more specifically. Instead of asking "How are you (physically)?" I would have asked, "How is your heart feeling?" *Lori, 39, partner, breast*

▸ I wish I had talked to her more about all that was going on. In order to cope better, I "intellectualized" her situation. I was only emotional when away from her. *Martha, 50, mother, non-Hodgkins lymphoma*

▸ You try to do the best you can each day, keeping up with your own family and children, comforting mom, taking care of myself, going to work. *Georgia, 48, father, lung*

▸ I feel that once the diagnosis was made, I gave everything I had to give. *Rosemary, 66, sister, ovarian*

▸ I do feel each of us did all we could physically, emotionally and financially to make sure his final days were comfortable. *Mary, 42, father, lung*

▸ Nothing, except maybe take better care of myself. *Darrell, 54, wife, lung*

▸ Been a better friend before the diagnosis. *Phyllis, 59, friend, prostate*

▸ Shared more of their fears, let them see me cry instead of showing a brave face. *Vera, 73, several relatives*

▸ I wish I could have taken more time off work, but was single at the time and couldn't afford to. *Tracy, 47, mother, lung*

▸ I wish I could have talked more about it and asked more questions. *Laura, 44, aunt, lymph*

▸ No, I was pregnant at the time and no one ever expected me to have a baby, so it gave Mom a purpose to go on. She had her last chemo on the day my son was born. *Carlene, 51, mother, breast*

▸ She was the most courageous person I ever knew. Depression set in when she knew there was no hope. It was the hardest thing to watch and feel so helpless to do anything but feel rage at the unfairness in my solitude. I wish I could have taken her place. The only salvation I have is knowing it would have been as unbearable for her if the roles were reversed. I don't think she could have taken it. *Annamarie, 62, daughter, NA*

▸ Started talking more openly sooner. The last four and a half months we were open and honest with each other. She shared her deepest concerns. *A loved one*

▸ Yes, talk more about "what ifs," family (we did a lot of that) and what he wanted. He had a lot of faith and he leaned on that. *Lynn, 64, brother, colon*

▸ I wish I would have spent more time with him. I wish I could have done something to save him. *Monica, 35, husband, pancreatic*

▸ Been more physical in showing love, i.e. hugs, kisses, holding his hand. Verbally expressing feelings toward him. *Edith, 65, husband, melanoma*

▸ Just having her come out alive and be a five-year survivor, you forget little things. *Liz, 43, sister, breast*

> "I wish I had said 'I love you' more often. We knew the love was there, but we didn't say it often enough."
> Lois, 53, mother, breast

▸ I think we've been very supportive. It is just a daily challenge to live with. *Patti, 52, husband, renal cell cancer*

▸ Would've kept in closer touch when recurrence took place. Was probably respecting privacy too much. *Ann, 51, friend, brain*

▸ To probe more when Dad was initially diagnosed. The end of his life with cancer was short, two weeks from diagnosis of full-blown internally to death. *Krista, 39, father, prostate*

▸ I wish I would have shared more with her, both my feelings for her and about the rest of my life. *Chris, 38, mother, breast*

▸ Nothing, except being at the hospital the morning of the day she died. *Barbara, 66, both parents*

▸ Even though we spent a lot of time together, I would have spent more. We talked a lot, but again, I would have talked more. *Mark, 45, wife, breast*

▸ I sometimes wished I would have just gone up to her and made her tell me if she needed to talk or needed me to do anything for her. That she could have depended on me more. *Barb, 44, best friend, non-Hodgkins lymphoma*

▸ I wish I would have not been so reserved offering physical help. I was afraid of stepping on her husband's toes or making her do something when she was too tired. *Susan, 49, best friend, lymphoma*

▸ More time in general. Been able to help with the head shaving and other things she tried to have fun with. Even shaved my own head with her. Too much. *Kathleen, 24, mother, breast*

▸ I wish it hadn't taken cancer to bring us closer. *Monica, 52, sister, NA*

▸ We wish we had done more. We counted on her adult children to be there and do more than they were willing to do. *Sharon, 65, friend, breast*

▸ I needed to have my own support system/friends where I could express what I couldn't say to my wife. Guys don't network this way like women do. *Paul 53, wife, breast*

▸ I would have been with her the night before she died. I was so stressed. I went out to a special dinner. *Nancy, 67, mother, pancreatic*

▸ Been a better listener. Shouldn't have downplayed some issues that seemed to be more important to him than me. *Peggy, 53, husband, prostate*

▸ I wish we would have gone to some counseling after the first time we heard those words. *Michael, 50, wife*

Loved ones say...

Looking back, what do you wish the patient would have said or done differently?

A loved one inquired as to why we asked this question on the survey, wondering if it came across perhaps a bit negative, putting an undue expectation on the patient. We thought that this was an appropriate companion question to the previous one, asking what the loved one would have said or done differently with the benefit of hindsight. The responses to both are quite revealing as most point out issues with communication and how expressing needs is crucial. The relationship between everyone touched by cancer and how to enhance that bond is the focus of this book.

▸ I wish my dad would tell my mom that he doesn't constantly want to talk about his cancer. She wants to and needs to, he doesn't. I'm trying to figure out how to tell my mom to "cool it" without offending her. *Laura, 44, father, prostate*

▸ Talked about what was happening. *Julie, 51, father, lung*

▸ No, he was just who he was, a good person, who would ask nothing of anyone, but give everything of himself to help others. *Georgia, 48, father, lung*

▸ Been more intent on asking or looking into what to expect, how soon to expect the end. *Virginia, 66, husband, colon; mother-in-law, colon*

▸ Been more active in the care of himself. Taken responsibility for his health and care rather than leave it to a pill or scalpel. *Judith, 70, husband, colon*

▸ I was the one who needed to change, not her. *Martha, 50, mother, non-Hodgkins lymphoma*

"I read and learned about treatment options and how treatments affect the patient." *Lois, 53, mother, breast*

▸ I wish she had gone to the doctor earlier. *Rosemary, 66, sister, ovarian*

▸ I wish he would have stopped smoking in 1980 or earlier instead of 1986. *Barbara, 66, husband, larynx*

268

▸ Allowed more help in the home sooner. *P, 66, sister-in-law, lung and bone*

▸ I wish she would have rested more. *Laura, 44, aunt, lymph*

▸ No, she did everything that was ever recommended or even suggested. *Carlene, 51, mother, breast*

> "Accepted his illness and faced his fear and shared them with us so we could help." Linda, 62, husband, colon

▸ He knows he did it his way, but I wish he would have gone to a big hospital for a transfusion sooner and not on a weekend. *Abbie, 51, father, leukemia*

▸ Been less critical of his situation. He just couldn't eat, and I tried so hard to find something he would like. I didn't know how sick he was. *Lynn, 64, brother, colon*

▸ Taken her pain meds on schedule. She sometimes thought the pain was gone without keeping the meds on schedule. Ouch! *Rue, 29, mother, breast*

▸ Talked more about his feelings, but he was never good about verbalizing his feelings. *Rose, 70, husband, lymphoma*

▸ To begin with, he was very appreciative. As his good health continued, he could be very cocky and say, "You've never really had to be a caregiver, etc." I'm not sure if he realizes this has affected his whole family. *Patti, 52, husband, renal cell cancer*

▸ Been more willing to share the pain of loss. *Chris, 51, friend, breast*

▸ I wish she had increased the pain patch sooner. *Linda, 65, best friend, breast*

▸ Took things slower and not belittle herself about how slow she thought she was, and always feeling bad about feeling bad. *Beverly, 50, best friend, mesothelioma*

▸ Told us the truth early on. *Krista, 39, father, prostate*

‣ Been more compliant. *Barbara, 66, both parents*

‣ Nothing. I have never seen anyone fight so hard, do what was asked of them, and maintain her dignity like she did. She inspired a lot of people. *Mark, 45, wife, breast*

‣ I wish he could have spoken about his feelings more. It may have helped him. He handled it the best way he could. *C, 63, father, esophageal and liver*

269

‣ I wish she would have depended on me more. *Barb, 44, best friend, non-Hodgkins lymphoma*

‣ At the time, I wanted her to be more realistic and act more worried and so then I could help more. But now, I'm so glad she did everything the way she did. *Kathleen, 24, mother, breast*

‣ She did this thing with grace. She did read a great deal about positive attitude, and felt guilty if she couldn't always maintain it! *Sharon, 65, friend, breast*

‣ A few more thank you's would have helped at certain times. *Michael, 50, wife*

"I love that my mom was very positive throughout the whole thing, but I wish she would have expressed her fears a little more openly. Then we all would have been able to help more." Maureen, 23, mother, breast

What I wish

What can I/we do differently now?

What I wish I would have done differently _____

_____

_____

What I wish my spouse/significant other would have done differently

_____

_____

What I wish my parents would have done differently _____

_____

_____

What I wish my children would have done differently _____

_____

_____

What I wish other loved ones would have done differently _____

_____

_____

What I wish my friends would have done differently _____

_____

_____

Survivors say...

What one thing helped you the most during diagnosis, treatment and recovery?

▸ When my friends and family all said they would be there for me. *V, 64, breast*

▸ A friend came to the hospital after my surgery, while still in ICU, and just listened and prayed. *Diana, 46, lung*

▸ Sense of humor. *S, 61, breast*

▸ Faith, prayer and my husband. I have not recovered. The chemo treatments caused great damage. They had to stop treatments. *Elaine, 72, leukemia*

▸ Being numb and I thought I was going to die. I felt I had no one so to me it didn't matter. *Donna, 72, colon*

▸ Trust, lots of trust. *Maria, 61, breast*

▸ Love and support of spouse. *Jim, 50, thyroid*

▸ My own strength. *N, 80, breast*

▸ Several dear friends with cancer came to tell me what had helped them, wonderful. *B, 93, breast*

▸ Determination. I was needed. *Muriel, 83, breast*

▸ Power of prayer by everyone. They supported me when I couldn't. *Judy, 56, breast*

▸ Nurses, doctors, God and friends. *Lois, 69, colon*

▸ Feeling that someone cared and prayer. Exercise. *Yvonne, 74, breast*

▸ All the people at the oncology unit. *Sandy, 58, breast*

▸ Knowing that the treatments would end, trusting in my doctors. *Marilyn 70, adenoid cystic carcinoma*

▸ Prayers from family, friends and people I didn't even know who had my name on their prayer chains. *Mary, 52, breast*

▸ Time. Not being given expectations to achieve. *V, 66, breast*

▸ My husband's positive attitude. *Robin, 46, breast*

▸ The kindness of the nurses and my doctor, and my best friend, who called and came by every day. *Alveretta, 85, ovarian*

▸ Determination that no matter how long I lived, I would live each moment and each day to the fullest. Death does not scare me. *Robert, 70, lung*

▸ Cards, friends visiting, preparing food. *Kathy, 61, breast*

▸ Friends closing ranks, cards of encouragement. Meals. They made me realize that I wasn't going through it alone. I never knew how much others cared. *Theresa, 49, breast*

▸ Faith and taking one moment at a time. *Gresha, 47, breast*

▸ I put myself in God's hands. Also I decided to look at it as sort of an adventure. Emotionally, I was at peace with it. *Rita, 58, breast*

▸ Having my wife with me. Being at home. *Bill, 64, throat, tongue*

▸ To be able to tell someone exactly how I felt knowing I would not be judged. Having my doctor gave me complete confidence. He was there for me 24/7. He gave me his home phone number! *Paula, 53, uterine and breast*

▸ Trying to carry on as normal as I could and having people understand that you need time to relax, and the cancer patient has to understand they can't do it all. *Nancy, 57, non-Hodgkins lymphoma*

▸ My 8 and 5-year-old children. I did not want them to see me as a quitter. *A survivor*

▸ Meeting women my age who were breast cancer survivors. *Noreen, 49, breast*

▸ Nature, being with children in normal situations, continuing my life. *Christine, 51, breast*

▸ My family and my job. As a caregiver, my residents needed my help and being there for them was helping me cope with cancer. It's like "who was holding whose hand." *Vicki, 53, breast*

▸ People who would listen to me and encourage me. *Shari, 50, breast*

Hey, I'm still fighting!

"I have been in remission one year. People seem to have forgotten that I am still going through tests." Tracy, 33, cervical

"No one said too much. I worked more than 40 hours a week. Many seemed to act as though the experience was done way before the treatments ever were." Joseph, 25, Hodgkin's lymphoma

"My family did not want to do support groups. Only last year did they visit me at the Relay for Life. The 'other' said, 'You HAD cancer, you don't now, move on.' We have no relationship." Diana, 46, lung

Some of the realities

▸ It's going to make the caretaker very angry, tired, overworked and resentful. *Pat, 57, husband, brain*

▸ I decided not to waste my time on some people who could not be truly counted on as friends. Life is too short. *Jeannie, 60, breast*

▸ Let people know that you don't have to be afraid of a cancer patient. It's still the same person they were before cancer. *Monica, 52, sister*

▸ Unfortunately, not all cancer patients have a strong faith, a strong family and a large network of compassionate friends scattered throughout the world. *Roger, 56, and Char, 59, friend, prostate*

▸ Tried not to take any rejection personally. *Peggy, 53, husband, prostate*

▸ Whatever emotions you're feeling, let them out. Holding your emotions in is very harmful. *Norma, 56, mesothelomia*

▸ Everyone reacts differently. We can't control others. Hopefully they will be supportive, but sometimes they have their own demons to confront. *Theresa, 49, breast*

▸ Someone needed me. *Muriel, 83, breast*

▸ Who's coping: me or them? *John, 55, wife, breast*

▸ Tell them it is OK to cry. *Theresa, 49, breast*

▸ She was hopeful and determined. How could we be any less? *Susan, 49, best friend, lymphoma*

▸ Re-connecting with family and friends to heal old wounds. *Mary, 52, husband, kidney*

▸ Always be yourself. The cancer patient doesn't want you acting like someone they don't know. They need stability at an unstable time. *Barb, 44, best friend, non-Hodgkins lymphoma*

▸ Caregiver may suffer as much as the patient. *Paul 53, wife, breast*

▸ Sometimes I believe it is harder for persons closest to you than you yourself. They feel helpless. *Helen, 71, NA*

Facing death

"I expect to pass through this world but once; any good thing therefore that I can do, or any kindness that I can show to any fellow creature, let me do it now; let me not defer or neglect it, for I shall not pass this way again." Ettiene De Grellet

Just one of many

276 End of life

If your friend does get a bad prognosis and comes closer to the end of life, they may need you more than at any other time. Some people are so afraid of death that they will pull away, especially when things become worse and death seems to be imminent. So many lessons can be learned near death by the way your friend deals with this. It is possible to gain so much if you do not pull away.

Not all, but many, people get a sense of clarity or calm near the end of life that can help others deal with their impending grief. The more you love your friend, the more you will miss them, but also, the more you can gain from them at this time. In American culture, death is thought of as failure by some and feared by many. Even though a large majority admit they believe in God in some form, that doesn't always help letting go of someone you love. We have learned that holding on to spiritual strength is very important at this time. Belief that your friend will always be there for you and will now be just in a "spiritual" form rather than a physical form can help.

Even if the process of death brings out anger in your friend, rather than calm, you will still have much to offer at this time. Assuring them they will always be loved and remembered can help so very much. Just being there to listen throughout the process of dying is more helpful than anything else. It is easy to be afraid and pull away, but keeping a strong bond until the end could be a very powerful and healing experience.

We are all human and will have many emotions at this time, such as fear, frustration and anger. These are necessary to acknowledge but don't let them interfere with your relationship and deprive you both of the experience you can gain by helping your friend get through this difficult time.

If we truly believe in God, death is not an end but a transition to something better. This is much easier to reflect on when you are not in the midst of this experience. Reminding your friend of heaven, praying with them and for them will help you both immensely.

Robin

277

Talking about death

Death.

It's the topic most of us avoid for good reason. However, it's a reality all of us must face, and losing a loved one is one of the most traumatic events of life.

Our questionnaire for survivors and loved ones didn't even have a specific question about the subject of death. Many volunteered their thoughts and how they were affected by the potential or actual loss of a loved one.

▸ The night he died I helped the nurse take him from the ER to his room, and I wish I had kissed him and said goodbye. I didn't think he would die so quickly. *Abbie, 51, father, leukemia*

▸ My sister said my husband and I got together so he could help me figure out how to live and for me to help him figure out how to die. *Mary, 52, husband, kidney*

▸ I was always there for him, he died in my arms. I drove him to doctor's appointments, gave him shots, medicine, IV feedings, got anything he asked for. I tried to never have him to be alone at treatments, hospital, etc. I told him I loved him and tried to be positive and give him hope. *Monica, 35, husband, pancreatic*

▸ Just being available to listen. She wanted everything in order as her death got closer. We talked about her funeral. *Mary, 63, best friend, breast*

▸ Sharing with her how much she had meant to me. *P, 66, sister-in-law, lung and bone*

▸ I was there with him the last two months, a lot. Emotionally we were very close, my older brother, and I never wanted to cry in front of him. *Lynn, 64, brother, colon*

"He knew that I would 'be there' for Mom after he died and that I would take care of things." *Abbie, 51, father, leukemia*

- I wish I'd have been more blunt and honest with his wife. I wish she would have realized he was dying. *Shirley, 66, brother, lung*

- I wish I had turned off the fan so I could have heard her last words to me. *Linda, 65, best friend, breast*

- I wish I would have been more patient in the end. *Lisa, 40, husband, brain*

- I wish I could have drawn out his feelings more. I didn't know how. That might have helped him to talk about it. *C, 63, father, esophageal and liver*

279

- I only wish he hadn't chosen to stay in denial until it was too late. *Linda, 62, husband, colon*

- (I wish he hadn't) shut himself off from me, but I think now that he had to do it to separate and begin the "letting go" process. *Mary, 52, husband, kidney*

- Looking back, it was a beautiful experience, and she told me she would let me know in little ways that she's always with me (and has). *Tracy, 47, mother, lung*

  "Dad seemed to smile more at everyone, his way to comfort us." *Georgia, 48, father, lung*

- What happens when your life is no longer anything but getting through the day. The overwhelming guilt of not doing enough. I held my daughter in my arms as she died. She was only a skeleton by then. I wanted to climb in the coffin with her and just hold her forever. *Annamarie, 62, daughter, NA*

- (I wish) for people not to be afraid to visit someone dying. Even if you don't know what to say, just being there shows you care. *Tracy, 47, mother, lung*

- I respected the way she lived with her disease. I wish her family could have talked with her about her death. *Mary, 63, best friend, breast*

- I wish he would have hugged me, kissed me, held my hand more. He felt unattractive, and the medications and pain made him unable to be sexually intimate, so I lost most of our intimacy long before he died. I wish we would have talked about a new relationship for me if he were to die. I wish he would have told me to love again and be happy. *Monica, 35, husband, pancreatic*

▸ I wish he could have shared his feelings about his illness and dying. *Shirley, 66, brother, lung*

▸ (I wish she had been) more specific of what to find and where to find things and her wishes after she passed. *Leonard, 41, wife, breast*

▸ He taught me that it was possible to die with dignity. *Lisa, 40, husband, brain*

▸ She came to acceptance more easily so we could talk about the reality of dying. *P, 66, sister-in-law, lung and bone*

▸ My wife had been a widow at age 23. Before she died, I wish she would have acknowledged the possibility of death, and talked with me about how to carry on. *Paul 53, wife, breast*

▸ We didn't discuss death until a little the last week. She let me know when I was present during a phone conversation to my niece, in which she said, "I won't be here in 10 days." *Nancy, 67, mother, pancreatic*

▸ I'm sad that our paths naturally diverged in focus when he chose to accept death and I began trying to figure out how to live without my best friend. *Mary, 52, husband, kidney*

▸ (I wish we had) talked more especially when her condition was terminal, talk about death. *Rudy, 81, wife, leukemia*

▸ (I wish I had) been able to talk about death better. The stress is incredible. Some family members do "run away" and will fail to help. You will be disappointed in them. *Nancy, 67, mother, pancreatic*

> "She handled it beautifully. She never complained, neve[r] said 'why me?' Just playe[d] the hand she was dealt."
> *Hiles, 69, wife, uterine*

▸ I wish I would have told him now much it would hurt to lose him. Maybe insisted on a different place for treatment. *Colleen, 60, husband, colon*

▸ Have no regrets. Say the important things. Do what the patient and you need to reach peace. *C, 63, father, esophageal and liver*

▸ No, she refused to talk about cancer or dying. *James, 55, mother, colon*

▸ Spend as much time together as possible. Discuss the future. Plan such things as pall bearers, purchase grave, marker, funeral music. Go through everything together. *Hiles, 69 wife, uterine*

▸ I wish that people would allow me to grieve as I do and not tell me to be quiet when I talked about the hours before Dad died. *Abbie, 51, father, leukemia*

▸ Mother gave us four children her treasures and told the stories about them, i.e., great-grandmother's cut glass bowl. She prepared us for her death. *Kay, 65, mother, leukemia*

▸ Yes, often speaking of heaven and how much better she will be when she sees Jesus face to face. *Kathleen, 49, friend, breast*

▸ We both knew what the outcome was going to be. She didn't want to die. *Annamarie, 62, daughter, NA*

▸ We didn't really talk about it. She was told she had two to three months to live. She was able to live longer and a fairly good life. *Nancy, 67, mother, pancreatic*

▸ When someone dies of cancer, please do not say, "It was a blessing" because no one wants it to be considered a blessing that he or she is gone. *Diane, 47, breast*

"Once Mom hugged me when I cried, and she said, 'We'll be together again someday.'"
Kay, 65, mother, leukemia

Anticipated vs. unanticipated grief

Anticipated grief occurs when there is knowledge or "anticipation" of an impending loss. This type of loss occurs when a cancer patient is terminal, or when there is recurrence of the cancer, coupled with a poor prognosis. Research has indicated that anticipatory grief has different elements than grief from a sudden loss.

With a sudden loss, the grievers tend to have difficulty with the full psychological, emotional, spiritual, and physical loss of the loved one. Sudden loss tends to turn your life upside down, and it is difficult to make sense of the loss, except from an intellectual perspective. In comparison, with anticipatory grief, the grievers have time to say good-bye, prepare for the impending death, deal with issues of changes in the family structure, the loss of companionship, and the fears related to death and dying. The grieving process may be the same for both types of grief, but with anticipatory grief, the grievers have time to "let go" and prepare for the impending death.

The National Cancer Institute states there are four typical issues, which occur in anticipatory grief:

▸ There is a greater emphasis and focus on the dying person.

▸ There is a "rehearsal" of the death...or a focus on the preparation for the death.

▸ There is deeply felt grief and depression.

▸ There is an attempt to find ways to cope with the impending death.

While there is a preparation period with anticipated grief, there is also the difficult task of "holding on" versus "letting go" of the loved one. In many cases, this is a challenging balance for caregivers and loved ones. Emotions pull the grievers in all directions and it's hard to find calm in the struggle.

Here are some tips for those dealing with anticipatory grief:

▸ Use journaling to sort out your feelings.

▸ Solicit and utilize a strong support network.

▸ Do things now, instead of waiting. Remember that chores can be done later, and nothing is more important than focusing on doing what you want with your time remaining together.

▸ Spend time with loved ones and supportive friends.

- Seek spiritual assistance or professional counseling, which can assist with grief and loss if you have difficulty finding a balance.
- Make preparations that will assist with the "rehearsal" process. Organize the funeral, prepare the obituary, talk about the service, discuss living wills, and prepare a plan for death with dignity and respect.
- Say "I love you" and find ways to heal any unfinished business.
- Accept your feelings of sadness, confusion, anxiety, and loss. These are all natural emotions and embrace your humanness.

283

How can I prepare for death?

How patients can say goodbye

- Notes to loved ones placed in envelopes
- Pre-recorded audio tapes
- Pre-recorded CDs

- Verbalize love
- Pre-recorded camcorder tapes
- Items to be opened at a later date
- Journals (*Note: please remember these can be delicate in nature*)
- Put aside gifts for children
- Put aside gifts for loved ones
- Letters for loved ones and friends pre-written
- Cards to be read at death
- Talk about expectations and desires at death
- Talk about funeral arrangements
- Create something to be read at the funeral or visitation
- Letters written to physicians, nurses, or other healthcare workers
- Hope chest for loved ones
- Perform a religious ceremony of "last rites"
- Having all legal documents, living wills, do not resuscitate orders, pill lists compiled
- Photo albums made of favorite memories
- Remember there is no "right way" to say goodbye

How loved ones can say goodbye

- Visit the cemetery and "talk" to loved one
- Take notes or keepsakes with you on trips or when away from home
- Have a necklace with vile of "ashes" made to wear
- Go to your church or synagogue and participate in the "mourners's prayers"
- Talk about happy memories

- Light a memorial candle on the anniversary of the death
- Light candles at your church
- Reassure the patient the family will be okay after the death
- Reassure the patient that wishes for the children will be accomplished after death
- Verbalize love to each other
- Keep picture of loved one in your pocket or purse
- Write a letter of love and appreciation to the patient
- Discuss what will happen after death and expectations for the future
- Give answers that will calm the patient at death
- Give permission to "let go" and die in peace and with dignity
- Remember there is no "right way" to say goodbye
- Attend a grief support group in your area

Saying goodbye

Forgiveness can be a key to healing

Learning to forgive is a valuable gift for your own emotional and physical health. Holding on to anger, resentments, and the related pain can manifest symptoms, which are harmful for the griever.

Those who have lost a loved one may have difficulty forgiving. Many times, grievers are angry at physicians, the hospital and helping professionals after the loss of a loved one. Sometimes people are also angry at themselves for not doing things (blaming themselves for not insisting on a second opinion, feeling like they had control to change outcomes). Additionally, some grievers feel anger and resentment directed towards the deceased for "leaving them."

It is important to remember that the "act of forgiving" doesn't mean condoning what happened or forgetting the offenses. Forgiveness means coming to a point where you can let go of some of the anger and pain, in a healthy manner. Research indicates that those who learn to forgive witness a decrease in symptoms such as headaches, stomach aches, backaches, depression, and other recurrent effects.

What are typical techniques for teaching forgiveness? The most common technique is writing a letter to the person who you believe has hurt you in some fashion. This letter is an open expression of all of your feelings, no matter how intense the feelings may be. It is important to understand that this letter is a form of a "good-bye" and it is used as a means of releasing emotions that have been locked deep within. Commonly, this letter can be read at a graveside, read in front of a picture, or read out loud; then tearing up the letter as a process of "letting go."

Another technique includes writing your painful feelings and then imagining that you are placing those feelings inside a balloon that is being sent out into the universe. This technique is an effective means of letting go of destructive thoughts.

Additional suggestions include talking to a licensed mental health therapist, a professional hospice counselor, attending a grief support group, or talking to your priest, rabbi or minister.

"With the medical profession-als, be adamant, be assertive, be strong, stand up at the time of death. It's important to be honest about what's going to happen and when it's going to happen. Say to those who helped the patient along the way, 'You don't need to come to the visitation. You don't need to come for me, but only if you need to come for your closure, since you've been there since day one.'" L, wife, breast

"What lies behind us and what lies before us are tiny matters compared to what lives within us."
Oliver Wendell Holmes

Death: Talking to children

A parent or grandparent is going to die … but how do you tell children? The key elements are to be truthful and reinforce the importance of talking about our feelings.

Developmentally, children see death in different ways.

Preschoolers may talk about death, but they see it as reversible and temporary in nature. Six-to-10 year olds have a little more understanding of death, but believe that death only happens to the elderly. Ten-to-13 year olds see death as final, but many times have feelings of guilt, believing in some fashion they may have caused the death to occur.

Dealing with the death of a parent due to cancer, children need to be reassured their basic physical and emotional needs will be met in an ongoing way, even if the loved one is deceased. They also need support and reassurance that they will continue to have loved ones around them who will take care of them.

Here are some important tips:

▸ **Be honest.** Children can sense something is wrong, and need to know the truth so they can mentally and psychologically cope.

▸ **Be clear about the reality of "death."** Make sure that children understand that the survivor will not return, and that they will not be back living with them in the future.

▸ **Don't cover up the truth.** Children can sense lies and deception. If children are not allowed to know the reality of the impending death, it will only increase their fear and resentment.

▸ **Encourage openness.** Answer all questions and encourage your children to ask any question they may have unanswered.

▸ **Try to keep the children's routine somewhat consistent.** Staying with a routine, whether it's bedtime rituals or eating at a regular time, will help children adjust to the death.

▸ **Be open about your feelings.** It's important that you let children see you grieve. If they see you grieve, they will understand that it is acceptable to show their own grief as well.

▸ *Include the children in some form of the death ritual.* Allow children to be part of the funeral, write a goodbye letter which is placed in the casket, put flowers on the grave, or some active part that will assist in their ability to "let go" and grieve.

▸ *Access assistance from grandparents and close relatives as nurturers.* Children need to feel comforted and safe with family and friends.

289

▸ *Children may fear both parents will die.* Reassure them that no one knows when they will die, but that you will probably be there for them for a long time.

Children's reaction to death

Death of a loved one is a difficult transition for everyone. But, what many people don't realize is that young children react very differently than adults when a family member dies. Preschool and younger children typically view death as temporary and reversible. If adults have a hard time wrapping their mind around death, young children have greater difficulty because they watch television shows where people or animals are hurt and magically reappear. They believe people leave for a moment, just like they see on television, but developmentally they don't understand the concept of "forever."

What are some of the normal childhood responses to death in the family?

▸ *For weeks the child may believe the person is still alive, or will reappear*

▸ *The child may be fearful of attending the funeral*

▸ *Children are likely to display feelings of sadness for a long period of time*

▸ *The child may display anger in play, or be aggressive with playmates or friends*

▸ *The child may have some regression in behaviors such as bedwetting, or speaking in "baby-talk"*

▸ *The child might experience nightmares and have difficulty sleeping alone*

▸ *The child may appear irritable toward the surviving family members*

▶ *Children may have difficulty in school (acting out, lower grades)*

▶ *Children may not want to attend school or leave the surviving parent*

▶ *Consider how children will be affected by the death of a loved one in the hospital or at home.* If the cancer patient dies at home, will the child avoid that location or room out of fright or sadness? Call upon the expertise of hospice staff for guidance on dealing with your individual situation.

▶ *All children react differently to loss.* Don't expect all of them to react in the same way

Surviving relatives should spend as much time as possible with the child, making it clear that it is safe to show their feelings or talk about grief. It is important to tell the child they were not the cause of what happened, or that you can't wish someone dead. Additionally, relatives may need to repeatedly explain the concept of death and what happens to a person when they die, if appropriate, from a religious or spiritual perspective.

Relatives can also assist by creating a ritual to help children "let go" or say goodbye to the lost loved one. This might include drawing pictures, taking flowers to the gravesite. Many children also find it comforting to visualize talking to their loved one at any time, or that the loved one is an angel watching over them.

What are some of the danger signs that suggest a child may need some assistance from a mental health professional?

▶ Extended period of depression with loss in interest in daily activities

▶ Inability to sleep, loss of appetite, or fears of being alone

▶ Acting much younger for extended periods of time

▶ Excessively imitating the deceased person

▶ Withdrawal from family and friends

▶ Sharp drop in school performance or refusal to attend school

▶ Talk of suicide or wanting "to join" the deceased.

"The question is not whether we will die, but how we will live." Joan Borysenko

Grief and bereavement

Death is one cause for grieving, but many other forms of loss can initiate grief. For instance, when you or your loved one was diagnosed with cancer, you experienced a form of grief. Immediately, your mind began to grieve the potential loss of your loved one, or your own life. You began to grieve the potential loss of the future times together, or perhaps being able to do the things you once loved. Or, in the extreme of cases, the potential loss of your loved one to terminal cancer.

What are the typical phases of grieving?

▶ *Immediate reactions include numbness, disconnection, shock and disbelief.* Many times people feel emptiness, disorganization, and anxiety and depression. Those who lose a loved one commonly believe they see their lost loved one across the street or around a corner. Grievers are fueled by auditory or visual hallucinations which makes them worry that they are going crazy.

▶ *Acute responses in which sadness and despair are more prominent.* There are loss of appetite, sleeplessness, exhaustion and physical concerns. Grievers tend to ruminate about events of the illness and the death, as well as missed opportunities. There is also a fear of losing the integrity of the memories of the lost person. In this stage there may be anger at the hospital, the physician, or even the person who is deceased.

▶ *Working-through phase.* Feeling a continued sense of loss, the griever has lessening anguish and longing. After six months, there often is a resurgence of fresh grief, which tends to scare the griever. This is sometimes triggered by "firsts": the first holiday, the first birthday, the first new year, etc., without the person. Many times there is a painful confrontation of needing to go on alone.

▶ *Reorganization phase.* This stage is encompassed by the task of going on, living with new routines and resuming relationships. In general, grieving takes three or more years of adjustment, although there is some submission of grief from 6-12 months.

Grieving and bereavement can be complicated when there is a lack of social support, a past history of psychiatric care, unanticipated death, suicide, death of a child and an ambivalent relationship with the deceased.

What are some of the additional options available for those who are grieving?

▸ Psychotherapy to do grief work
▸ Psychopharmacology medications for limited usage for insomnia, major depression or reducing anxiety.
▸ Support groups through hospitals, cancer centers, churches, funeral homes, hospice, or organized bereavement groups.

Working through grief

▸ Accept your grief. It is important to give yourself the gift of allowing yourself to grieve
▸ Remind yourself that each stage of grief has a purpose
▸ Remind yourself that the grief will lessen with time
▸ Take care of your health (nutrition, sleep, exercise, etc)
▸ Process the loss with your support network
▸ Make time to be alone with your feelings
▸ Remind yourself that grief hurts, but it will not harm you
▸ Don't let others' expectations of grieving change your process
▸ Witness small moments when you focus on the future
▸ Ask for help from others, including a therapist

What are some tips for helping someone who is experiencing a major loss?

▸ Allow them to feel whatever they are feeling without shaming
▸ Don't push grievers into hiding their feelings or covering up their grief
▸ Just be there for those who are grieving. Please don't ignore or avoid them.
▸ Let them tell you about their loss again and again if needed. It is common for loved ones to speak of their pain repeatedly.
▸ Remember that grieving takes time. Many people say they notice a decrease in their grief within 3-5 years.
▸ Encourage grievers to seek help if they don't seem to be moving forward in the process

292

When no one can control this crazy world

Usually on top of the prayer list are prayers for good health, recovery and the destruction of cancer. However, also high on the list for patients/survivors and their loved ones is the need for someone to listen to them, especially if death is imminent. Those who can find the courage to talk about their experiences and feelings can learn from each other right up to the final breath.

Those who have worked with the dying often note that they receive far greater emotional rewards in return than they ever give in assistance. One counselor who works with cancer support groups notes that while it is gut-wrenching to observe, she has seen that hose individuals who communicate and open up their hearts and thoughts die with more grace and peace. Somehow they find an amazing courage after they've been allowed to express themselves and know that they've been heard.

It isn't easy, but cancer patients and those who love them can weather this journey better when they refuse to stop living even though they're dying. Those who savor every moment of life reinforce the concept that we can accomplish many great things in a very short period of time. A goal, a mission or a purpose can give the patient an unimagined boost of energy and resiliency when they understand the power of the mind over the body.

A huge value is placed on patients sharing experiences. An intimate group of a half dozen can be more beneficial to some than just attending a support group meeting. They can bond in a way that they can sustain each other and make those final moments and months more fulfilling for those who lose the battle, and leave survivors richer for having had this connection.

Hospice workers and counselors who witness this phenomenon are transformed by the power of those they help, those they see leave all their pain and suffering behind upon death.

We can all learn a lesson from those who comprehend the true meaning of life ... being with and embracing those we love.

Kathleen: Affecting my life in a profound way

294

By Joy Erlichman Miller, Ph.D.

When she entered my life, I knew there was something I was destined to learn from this woman. During the three years we knew each other, she was struggling with breast cancer. She would valiantly proclaim she would "beat this thing" because she had to stay alive for her two girls. If anyone could beat cancer, I believed it was going to be her. Standing like a cheerleader, I kept telling her she could beat this disease, while both of us knew that the chances were quite slim.

Every time we met, I knew we both were being transformed through our connection. I taught her techniques aimed at resiliency, and she taught me about gratitude. Upon reflection, I guess we taught each other to be resilient and the importance of being grateful for each moment we have on this earth.

I was there when she died, and I believe we both knew we had done all we could ... There was a deep sense of awareness that my life was profoundly changed forever because of this amazing woman.

As I write this book I remember her smile, her unbelievable strength, her dedication to her purpose, the devotion to her children, and the lesson of living each moment as if it was your last.

I know my story is not unique. Many of us lose people due to cancer. But, do we take time to learn life lessons ... or do we blindly close our eyes and just move on?

I remember after she died I received one of those computer stories and I've kept it for all these years on my computer. I don't know who wrote the original story, but I know these held important lessons to remember ...

Sometimes people come into your life and you know right away that they were meant to be there, to serve some sort of purpose, teach you a lesson, or to help you figure out who you are or who you want to become. You never know who these people may be (possibly your roommate, neighbor, co-worker, long-lost friend, lover, or even a complete stranger), but when you lock eyes with them, you know at that very moment they will affect your life in some profound way.

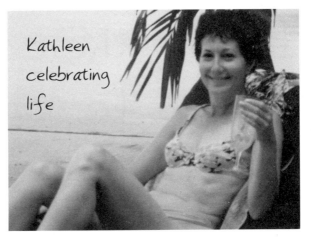

Kathleen celebrating life

And sometimes things happen to you that may seem horrible, painful, and unfair at first, but in reflection you find that without overcoming those obstacles you would have never realized your potential, strength, willpower, or heart. Everything happens for a reason. Nothing happens by chance or by means of good luck.

Illness, injury, love, lost moments of true greatness, and sheer stupidity all occur to test the limits of your soul. Without these small tests, whatever they may be, life would be like a smoothly paved, straight, flat road to nowhere. It would be safe and comfortable, but dull and utterly pointless.

The people you meet who affect your life, and the success and downfalls you experience, help to create who you are and who you become. Even the bad experiences can be learned from. In fact, they are probably the most poignant and important ones.

If someone hurts you, betrays you, or breaks your heart, forgive them, for they have helped you learn about trust and the importance of being cautious when you open your heart.

If someone loves you, love them back unconditionally, not only because they love you, but because in a way, they are teaching you to love and how to open your heart and eyes to things. Make every day count.

Appreciate every moment and take from those moments everything that you possibly can for you may never be able to experience it again. Talk to people that you have never talked to before, and actually listen.

Let yourself fall in love, break free, and set your sights high. Hold your head up because you have every right to. Tell yourself you are a great individual and believe in yourself, for if you don't believe in yourself, it will be hard for others to believe in you. You can make of your life anything you wish.

Create your own life and then go out and live it with absolutely no regrets. Most importantly if you LOVE someone tell him or her, for you never know what tomorrow may have in store. (Author unknown)

The choice is yours … do you integrate this message into your life in this moment … or do you turn the page and move away from the life lesson presented to you?

Finding the courage to talk to someone who is dying

By Monica Vest Wheeler

In November 1999, I spent more than a week with my in-laws in Florida, well aware that this might be the last time I would see my mother-in-law, Janice, alive. We all knew she was entering the final stages of a fatal disease, amyloidosis, sometimes associated with certain forms of cancer. For about eight years, she had battled it with the same vigor and feistiness she had exhibited all her life, at least in the life I had been privy to share since I first met her oldest son and her in 1974.

I will never forget that time I spent with her in late 1999. We talked and laughed as always. Our relationship had not changed, nor diminished as her physical strength ebbed away. Upon her request and to my delight, I took her out about every other day, the days when she had the energy to go, the moments when she insisted upon walking and pushing a cart instead of using a wheelchair.

"Thank you, honey, but I want to walk while I still can," she'd say, looking me in the eye. I'd almost start to protest because I worried about how she'd hold up, but wisely I shut my mouth. I couldn't deny her this simple pleasure.

She'd spend the days between our adventures recuperating as the toll continued to decimate her, her weight dropping by then to barely more than 100 pounds. Those were the days when she sat in the kitchen reading cookbooks, though her body couldn't tolerate any of the delights she savored on paper. I had my mess spread over her dining room table less than 10 feet away, working on the novels I hoped to publish one day.

However, I achieved nothing on paper except worthless scribbles. Instead, I spent hours, days, wasting time trying to work up the courage to ask Janice about life and death. I'd look up frequently and try to force the words, but my lips uttered nothing except, "Find any good recipes?"

I was afraid, not of her, but afraid to cry, afraid to show how fearful I was of losing her, instead anticipating the void her passing would leave in my life and not seizing these precious moments we now shared. So, I didn't ask the questions for the answers that my heart, mind and soul yearned to discover, the mysteries of life and death. My loss, my terrible, terrible loss, because I know she would have told me *if I had only asked.*

I had overheard her talk to my mother on the phone …

"I'd love to see you, too, but it's just not possible. I want you to remember me the way I was … I chose not to go back on chemotherapy. A life without quality isn't much of a life at all … My stomach has been destroyed by this disease, and my kidneys or heart will be next. I'm starting to have kidney problems now. Ivan (husband) knows what's happening. The kids know what's happening. I'm so glad Monica is here. She's always been so wonderful to me …"

I then cried, alone, in the bathroom.

One day, I watched her move about in frustration and finally slump into her thickly cushioned chair. I immediately went to her side and asked what she needed, mentally preparing for any medical emergency. Nothing, she said, breaking into tears I had never witnessed. She was outraged that her body couldn't do what she wanted it to. I just held her hand and let my tears fall with hers. After five minutes of silence, she sighed, signaling the end of the emotional crisis, "Okay, that's enough for today."

And it was. And I had let a moment of opportunity for a heartfelt conversation slip away. She returned to her cookbooks, and I went back to chastising myself for not speaking up.

When I said good-bye to fly back home, I just wrapped my arms around her, crying, still seeking the courage to say more than "I love you," to ask all the hows and whys that swirled viciously in my soul. I couldn't, even as I could feel every bone in her back and arms. I knew I'd never see her again.

At home, I regretted it almost obsessively for not speaking up. I still couldn't even though we talked on the phone three or four times a week. *Why couldn't I do it? Dammit!* I cursed myself.

In early February 2000, I started to write Janice a letter that grew day by day, thanking her for everything she had given me, how her son and I had grown closer as our marriage matured. I may have not asked *the* questions, but I made it clear how much she meant to me. I took the 14-page letter to the post office and mailed it on Friday, February 11.

On Saturday, February 12, she died.

She never got the letter. It was waiting for her, for me, when I arrived in Florida for her memorial service. The rest of the family thought I would want the unopened packet. I brought it back with me as a grim reminder of the consequences of postponing my priorities and letting ridiculous fears rob me of precious moments.

I hated myself.

It was more than a year later, after considerable internal grieving and beating myself up, that I sat down and wrote Janice another letter. This time, she was reading it over my shoulder ...

There's not one memory of my life with you that I would trade. Well, maybe one. I wish I had talked to you more during that final visit. I was afraid to cry and that's why I couldn't bring myself to talk to you. I sacrificed much, all in the silly name of saving myself from a red, blotchy face by not crying.

If I could have physically handled it, I would have cried much of that week, those 10 days. I feared migraines, loss of self-control. My God, that pain was a featherweight compared to the discomfort and agony you endured every day. Then again, maybe if I had allowed myself to cry, I would have gotten it all out of my system in the first few days and then allowed my soul to reach out to you.

And what would I have talked to you about? I remember sitting

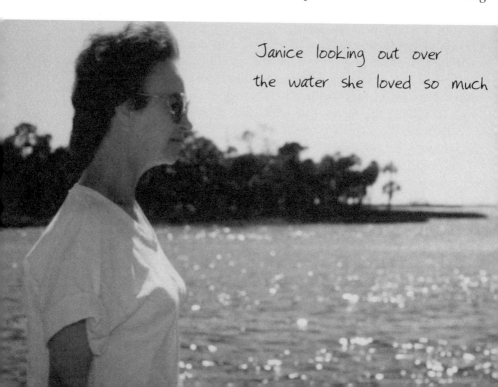

Janice looking out over the water she loved so much

there at your kitchen table with my papers and you there in your cush-
ioned chair about eight feet away, book in hand and absorbed. I looked
up several times, searching for the courage to ask such invasive, yet ten-
der questions like:

▸ *What goes through your mind every day?*
▸ *What does it feel like to know you're dying?*
▸ *What would you give anything to see? Taste? Touch? Smell? Hear?*
▸ *How have you made "peace" with God?*
▸ *What are the greatest lessons you've learned about life?*
▸ *What would you have done differently?*
▸ *Does death frighten you?*
▸ *How do you know there's a God?*
▸ *What was it that you saw in me so many years ago that made you*
   love me?
▸ *Why did you take me under your wing?*
▸ *Why did you always make me feel so special?*
▸ *Did you see the deep pain in my eyes, the emotional and spiritual*
   misery I experienced while visiting you that last time?
▸ *Do you believe in destiny? In fate?*
▸ *Are you angry at what has happened to you?*
▸ *Do you know how much I love you?*

Now, would those have been silly questions, meaningless inquiries,
or food for a feast at a table of connected souls? I feel robbed that I did
not ask some or all of those questions, as some new ones have come to
me now ...

I keep that letter in my journal, a reminder of how little
effort, yet how much courage it takes to reach out from deep
within yourself. How do you talk to someone who's dying, a
person you love so much?

You don't need a script or an orator's voice.

You don't need a box of tissues. A shirt sleeve will sop up the
tears and runny nose just as well.

You only need love and compassion.

Now I know. Now I am not afraid.

That's what Janice would have said ... if I had only asked.

Wait. Now, I remember. I had posed *the* question when I told
her how I was going to make mimosas for friends of mine. I
asked if I should use fake champagne. She laughed.

"Use the real thing, honey. Live it up and enjoy life. Have
some fun."

299

Postscript

When we started this project and sent out the surveys, one for survivors and another for family and friends, we were amazed at the response. The overriding message was a need for the words, the simple tools to communicate better with our loved ones during this most difficult time. Here are just a few examples of what they hoped this book would do:

▶ Explain stages of feelings, i.e. denial, anger, acceptance.

▶ Give suggestions on coping with changes in attitudes and behaviors.

▶ Discuss the importance of maintaining a positive attitude.

▶ Discuss how important it is to treat people as you always have. Don't avoid or abandon them. Ask what would be most helpful. Don't assume.

▶ Explore the emotions that they went through because you feel so lonely.

▶ Talk about how humor, hope, straight talk, information to raise awareness.

▶ Offer information for spouses to understand the emotions and needs.

▶ Explain how cancer is not always fatal.

▶ Offer advice on how to assert yourself in expressing needs.

▶ Talk about acceptance and moving on.

▶ Discuss how to acknowledge the fear, push through it and talk about what is happening.

▶ Help us find ways to nurture ourselves to be more effective caregivers.

▶ Discuss how people feel when diagnosed, how they coped and reacted.

▶ Offer ways for caregivers to cope when overwhelmed by family and work obligations.

▶ Discuss ways to get patients to share and how to listen and respond with the right words.

▶ Talk about how "quiet" people who don't normally express their feelings, what could I do to break through to be of help?

▶ Talk about the importance of having a support system

▸ Things for friends/family to say/do and not say/do.
▸ How to take the most realistic approach to facing cancer.
▸ Dealing with death and the dying process.
▸ Hope and positive things that happen because of cancer.
▸ Understanding that there is more than "one way" to feel.
▸ Normalizing their feelings, emotions. Confirming that they are not alone. Ways to care for themselves while going through this.
▸ How to be positive in any negative situation. To act normal around a cancer patient, what to do when you're not sure what to do.
▸ How to treat a patient. What do they want to talk about? Do they want us to push them? What is the best caregiver approach?
▸ Tell people what the patient might really be thinking, as opposed to the brave face they put on for loved ones.
▸ How to cope with feelings of "running away" or being in denial. How to make patient feel better. What does she want to hear?
▸ Offer a comprehensive book so I could find myself in there somewhere.

301

It was very difficult to narrow down all the respondents' inspiring and insightful notations. This book could have been twice this size with all the feedback we got and new ideas that came up along the way. But we believe we've offered at least a starting point in answering these requests and initiating those conversations.

What was particularly sobering to us was also the realization that at least three of the survivors who responded to our survey lost their battle with cancer before this book was completed. Unfortunately, those were but three of the reasons we pushed ourselves to finish this volume.

This book may not be perfect, but it's been created with intense devotion, heart, soul, and emotional and physical energy. But we're only human. And that's why we encourage you to let us know what you think of the book and what we might add to future editions by dropping us a line on our website at *www.cancerhelpbook.com* or through the mail at BF Press, P.O. Box 3065, Peoria, IL 61612-3065.

We wish you the strength, courage and voice to battle this despicable enemy called cancer.

Special acknowledgements

We'd like to thank the following individuals for helping make this project a reality:

302

Fred & Tilley Allen
Duffy Armstrong
Peggy Ault
Kathy Burdon
Kathy Corso
Alison, Allen, Kathleen &
    Maureen Cullinan
Fred Dirkse
The Drazin family
Gina Edwards
Janet Frietsch
Genny Gibbs
Peggy Hasty

Michele Holman
Mary Lemons
Donna Mueller
Theresa Schieffer
Laura Sollenberger
Carol Tuttle
Leonard & Eileen Unes
Leonard "Lenny" Unes II
Evelyn Vogel
The staff & volunteers of the
    Cancer Center for Healthy
    Living, Peoria, Illinois

A special thank you to the more than 250 survivors, family members and friends who completed the surveys. Without you, this book would not have been possible.

And to our spouses for their love, patience & moral support: *John Miller, Roger Wheeler* and *Doug Oberhelman*.

For more information

For recommended reading, resources, websites or organizations, contact:
▶ Your local office of the American Cancer Society, call 1-800-ACS-2345 or go online at **www.cancer.org.**
▶ The National Cancer Institute, call 1-800-4-CANCER or online at **www.nci.nih.gov/**

Also check our BF Press website at **www.cancerhelpbook.com** where we welcome your feedback for future editions of this book.

This book does not make nor attempt to make any diagnosis or suggest any specific treatment regarding any personal physical or emotional health issues. Consult a certified professional to address any concerns.

Meet the authors

Joy Erlichman Miller, Ph.D.

An internationally known licensed psychotherapist, professional trainer and author of six published books, Joy Erlichman Miller, Ph.D., is a leading authority on relationships issues, Holocaust studies, and trauma resolution. Dr. Miller has appeared on the Sally Jessy Raphael, Oprah Winfrey, Jenny Jones, Montel Williams and Geraldo Rivera shows. She hosted her own radio show and presents a weekly mental health segment on a CBS television station. She is the founder of Joy Miller & Associates in Peoria, Illinois. Dr. Miller is an Illinois state Licensed Clinical Professional Counselor as well as a Certified Master Addictions Counselor. Additionally, she was a part-time instructor at Bradley University and a faculty member at Walden University in the doctoral psychology program. She and her husband, John, live in Peoria, and have a son, Josh.

303

Monica Vest Wheeler

A former weekly newspaper reporter and editor, Monica Vest Wheeler is a free-lance writer who focuses on personality features. A graduate of the University of Evansville, she has researched and written six Peoria, Illinois, area history books since 1994, covering topics from entertainment to medical, including *The Grandest Views* and *Beyond the Mountaintop: A History of the Itoo Society*. She has several more books in the works on a variety of subjects, including the Holocaust. The designer of this book, she also presents programs on Peoria history and writing. She lives in Peoria with her husband, Roger, and son, Gordo.

Diane Cullinan Oberhelman

A breast cancer survivor, Diane Cullinan Oberhelman is a commercial real estate developer in Peoria, Illinois, and has properties throughout the United States. She's chief operating officer of Cullinan Properties, Ltd. She's involved in a variety of charitable organizations, including Kids Konnected in Peoria, the support group for children whose parents have cancer. Diane resides near Peoria with her husband, Doug, and has four children, Kathleen, Maureen, Alison and Allen.

Cancer: Here's how YOU can help ME cope & survive

To order additional copies of this book

304

Use this form or order larger quantities online at
www.cancerhelpbook.com

The cost of each book is **$19.95**

Shipping and handling (S/H) per book is $7

Name _____

Address _____

City _____

State _____ Zip _____

Phone _____

E-mail _____

# of books _____ **x $19.95**   _____

# of books _____ **x S/H $7**   _____

Sales tax for Illinois residents 6%   _____

TOTAL ENCLOSED   _____

MAKE CHECK OR MONEY ORDER PAYABLE TO BF PRESS AND MAIL TO
BF Press, P.O. Box 3065, Peoria, IL 61612-3065

Please note that these above prices are in effect until 12/06.
After that date, please check our website www.cancerhelpbook.com
for any possible changes.